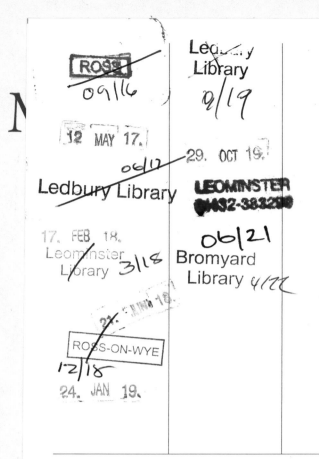
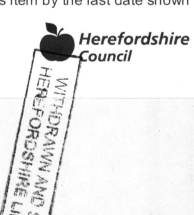

MESSAGE TO MY GIRL

*A dying father's
powerful legacy
of hope*

DR JARED NOEL

WITH DAVID W. WILLIAMS

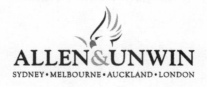

ALLEN&UNWIN

SYDNEY · MELBOURNE · AUCKLAND · LONDON

First published in 2015

Copyright © David Wyn Williams 2015

Allen & Unwin
Level 3, 228 Queen Street
Auckland 1010, New Zealand
Phone: (64 9) 377 3800

83 Alexander Street
Crows Nest NSW 2065, Australia
Phone: (61 2) 8425 0100
Email: info@allenandunwin.com
Web: www.allenandunwin.co.nz

A catalogue record for this book is available
from the National Library of New Zealand

ISBN 978 1 877505 54 6

Internal design by Kate Barraclough
Set in 13/16 pt Adobe Garamond Regular by Post Pre-press Group
Printed and bound in Australia by Griffin Press

10 9 8 7 6 5 4 3

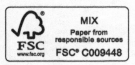

MIX
Paper from
responsible sources
FSC® C009448

The paper in this book is FSC® certified. FSC® promotes environmentally responsible, socially beneficial and economically viable management of the world's forests.

Contents

Breathing

I have a job that confronts life, death and everything in between.

I have a life that confronts living, dying and the reality of being in the middle.

I have patients who have to confront their own mortality in order to find their life.

Currently I work on the cardiothoracic ward at Auckland Hospital. We have people of all ages who have to go through what can only be described as major surgery, not without its risk, in order to squeeze more out of life. For some, they squeeze an extra five years; for others, the younger patients, they aim to squeeze another 50. Some are successful and, as I discovered in the first week of the job, some make great progress only to have their heart stop, and despite all efforts, not restart.

When life and death are so closely intertwined with day-to-day work, you can almost become desensitised to death. Death can become another statistic . . . and then I remember my diagnosis. I remember that I am going to become that statistic. I remember that behind that statistic is a life. One lived (hopefully) well, and one that hopefully dies well.

Then I remember that we are all dying. Ten out of ten people will die, we just do it at different rates; we do it unpredictably. Whether it is being hit by a bus, or being diagnosed with cancer, or passing away in our sleep in the distant future, we are all heading in the same direction.

And then I realise that while I might be at risk of desensitisation to death and dying, what I have noticed is that others are desensitised to being alive. Somehow, the value of life has been forgotten because medicine has been so good at hiding us from death.

Life for me has become a precious commodity, one that carries more value than any comparative analogy might offer. I know my life is short, but it is worth every second, and every breath, because they are breaths and seconds that I will never get to relive. I have seen too many people who have become desensitised to life, those for whom money, Apple products, ambition or self-interest retain more value than the breath they just took. Apple products are cool, but the breath I just took is what allows me to appreciate them; and the breath I just took has no value but for the grace of God who gives it to me.

And if I value my own breath so much, then it is a waste if it is not spent serving those who also breathe . . . otherwise I'm a self-serving fool.

'Life, death, and breathing', The Boredom Blog, June 22, 2011

Introduction

At the funeral of Dr Jared Noel on Monday, October 13, 2014, his friend and colleague Dr Paul Sharplin told a story about what he called Jared's 'cancer bombs', one-liners Jared was fond of using about his cancer as a way of making conversation with friends unbearably awkward. He was the consummate conversation stopper, drawing on his black humour to help him cope with the fact that he was dying, while also acting on his conviction that those around him should approach his condition with the same level of humour, honesty and humanity as he did himself.

For almost six years, from his initial diagnosis through to his death, Jared used words to help him face his illness with grace and nobility. He also used words to educate people on how to live well in the face of their mortality, and how to confront taboo subjects such as cancer, dying, suffering, love, faith and doubt—conversation stoppers Jared had a knack of turning into conversation starters. Soon after his diagnosis in November 2008, Jared began a blog that, by the time of his death, had attracted three-quarters of a million views. He began the blog initially to alleviate his boredom during rounds of chemotherapy, but it quickly became the means by which he kept friends and distant family members abreast of his condition. Ultimately, it became a didactic tool, challenging the taboos of death and dying with humour and unnerving honesty, and encouraging readers to recognise and treasure moments in life they would ordinarily take for granted. As Jared's readership grew, he wondered at the extraordinary turn his life had taken and the audience he had been given to share his thoughts with. This was a gift he never took for granted. His customary sign-off, 'Thanks for listening', was an authentic note of gratitude that gave Jared purpose until his very last days.

From one small post titled 'The birth of something new . . .' Jared's words became thoughts, his thoughts became blogs, the blogs became interviews, the interviews resulted in articles, the articles became conversations, and then, one day, the conversations ended. The ultimate taboo, death itself, brought an end to Jared's moment in the spotlight. But not before he impacted thousands of people with his inspirational message of living a full life in every moment while acknowledging and tackling head-on the brutal realities of that same life. In his final weeks, Jared became determined to record his reflections so the conversation could continue well after his own voice had ceased to play its part.

When I met Jared for the first time, on August 26, 2014, he was alone in a room in the West Auckland Hospice, sitting upright in bed and waiting for nothing in particular. Some weeks later, I discovered from his wife, Hannah, that this was a particularly difficult time for Jared, not just because he was preparing to die but because, in his words, he had nothing to do and nothing to say. His dream of putting his story together, primarily so that his baby daughter, Elise, might one day know her dad, was fading quickly. By his own estimate, he had no more than eight weeks to live.

I had known Jared for about eighteen months or so, but we had never met. I had seen him from time to time in my favourite café, which was owned and operated by a collective of which he was a member. Like others, I had followed his growing media profile and read his blog. What I liked about Jared's posts was his ability to speak about taboo matters with disarming and confrontational honesty but also, because he was a doctor, with clinical precision and pragmatism. His was a refreshing and healing approach to a heavy topic that had become very personal to me in the preceding twelve months.

The magazine I published at the time ran a small story when friends of Jared began a Givealittle crowdfunding campaign to raise money for a course of chemo treatment that would keep him alive long enough to meet his then unborn child. It was a remarkable campaign, and Jared's story had a great impact on the New Zealand public. The picture of Jared I had in my head when I fronted up to the hospice that day was the smiling, youthful face that had been published on the front page of the national newspaper, *The New Zealand Herald*. But the Jared I saw through the window of his closed hospice door, in the brief moment before he noticed my approach, looked nothing like that youthful, full-faced guy. He had a thick beard, thin, middle-aged hair, and wore glasses. His face had taken on a gaunt, malnourished look. I had seen him barely three months earlier looking totally different to this. Over the coming weeks I would look closely into Jared's face, trying to get beyond the beard and the glasses, to see if I could make out the guy from the pictures, the one I remembered. But I never did see him, and as time went on, he looked less and less like his old self.

In that first conversation, we mapped out a strategy for the development of this book. We talked every day until Jared felt that he could contribute nothing more. We concentrated on the interface between Jared's story and the big themes of the 'human drama' that he had begun to examine in his blog: love, marriage, fatherhood, faith, suffering, hope, mortality, purpose—the stuff of life. It had been Jared's goal for some time to write a book that expanded on these ideas, but time had beaten him. As he admitted to me, in the final few months of his life he got used to being a stay-at-home dad and did not want to concede any more time to cancer than he needed to, particularly when that time could be better spent with his daughter.

So we met daily, with the odd day off, until September 24. It was customary for me to text Jared to check that everything was okay before going to the house. On a small number of occasions he had cancelled at the last minute because he felt too sick. On this day, Jared did not cancel, but he did text this: 'Yep, but could be one of our last sessions. I'm still not doing great most days.' Our final conversation lasted some 50 minutes, and I never saw Jared again.

This book is a record of Jared's reflections on his incredible story and of the unique insight he developed into humanity's suffering as well as its hope. All of the content is taken from our conversations—21 in total, each one lasting about an hour. Material from Jared's blog is used where relevant, as this also formed a large part of our conversation. Each day we would discuss his condition, his ongoing hopes and what he feared, his growing awareness of mortality, his reflections on life, and his thoughts regarding the themes of his blogs. We also talked about the book's structure, its purpose and goals, what Jared hoped to achieve with it, and how he wanted to present his story. Some conversations were less like journalistic interviews and more like counselling sessions, as Jared processed many aspects of his impending death out loud, all of which is included in the final text. For me, it was a very 'sacred' time—an intimate engagement with the mind of a brilliant young man who was facing the biggest challenge of his life. And it was an act of incredible grace on Jared's part to give a stranger his story in his dying days and send him off with the words, 'I am just trusting you.'

This is Jared's story, told from Jared's perspective and in Jared's words. Although he never got the chance to write this material down himself, every word represents what he wanted to communicate to the world after he had gone. The final text is not a verbatim record of the conversations we had. The voice that speaks in what follows is, rather, a collaboration between the two of us—his reflections, his memories, his feelings, honed in the crucible of quite intense conversation in his final days, then put down in a final form by me. Jared got the opportunity to read a section before he died and responded with the words, 'It's perfect.' I am told that, from Jared, this is high praise indeed. To ensure that the final text is true to what Jared intended, his wife, Dr Hannah Noel, has been closely involved every step of the way.

Jared would speak often of his calling and his belief that he was meant to achieve great things on behalf of others. Life did not go as Jared planned, but he achieved great things nevertheless. And I know from experience the impact he had on those around him, even in—or perhaps because of—his illness. Ultimately, Jared worked to the very end so that Elise would have a picture of her dad. Ironically, he should not have been alive. He and I should never have met, and he should not have had the time to get his story down. Jared was alive because of an amazing outpouring of generosity by the New Zealand public, sparked by the impending birth of Elise and the great things Jared had achieved. It was the only reason he was alive. As Jared himself said to me, he would have died many months before but for Elise.

I had not realised how much I had been impacted by Jared personally until, a week before he died, I found myself in the emergency department with pancreatitis, and that night was told by a doctor there was a chance I would die from my illness.

I was in hospital for more than a week. On day six I went into surgery, and as I was being prepped I remember looking around the theatre, thinking of Jared, the work he did, and his singular approach to life that had dominated my thoughts during my hospital stay. I remember thinking how lucky I was that I was breathing, and how important that had suddenly become to me.

My surgery was successful. I was discharged on a Monday and went home to work on this book.

Jared died two days later.

David W. Williams
January 17, 2015

CHAPTER 1
Death on its own terms

What it essentially boils down to is that I am now waiting to die. I don't necessarily want to delay that for as long as possible. I'm not sure what I want, to be honest. I'm helpless at the moment. Death will come to me as quick or as slow as it decides, on its own terms.

'Palliative care 1.0', The Boredom Blog, August 30, 2014

It is the afternoon of Wednesday, September 24, 2014.

And I am dying.

I most likely will not die today or tomorrow. Next week perhaps. Or the week after. And while I very much want to live, if I am honest, death cannot come quickly enough. I am ready to go. Ready to be welcomed into the next phase of the journey, whatever it is.

I have been dying for almost six years, so I have had plenty of time to get used to the idea. But dying of a terminal illness is not like a steady decline to the end. It is a dynamic battle with possibilities, probabilities, inevitabilities. You are given bad news. Then worse news. Then you pick yourself up and decide to keep going, to keep holding on to your calling. And then you find some hope. And then the hope is dashed. And then a miracle occurs. But the miracle occurs in the context of a reality you can never fully deny. You are dying, and the end has to come some time.

For me, that time is now.

These extraordinary years will end here, in this room, where the family will gather around the bed to see me go. None of us know the day or the time—nature will take its course—but we know that it is soon.

And I am ready, apart from one, unfinished thing. Eight months ago, Elise came into my world under remarkable circumstances. The day she was born, I should not have been alive. My life was extended because a whole lot of people—some friends and family, but mostly people we had never met—did something extraordinary for us. For Elise. And because of that, on January 17, I delivered Elise, my daughter, who I thought I would never see. And moments later, when I got to hold her against my chest, the significance of that moment sank in. But I realised, some weeks after we brought her home and began family life right here, in this house, that I would die before she truly knew me. She has the photos, and she has the stories, and she can read almost six years' worth of blogs. But Elise will never know me. Never remember me.

And so the day that I came home to die, I determined to leave her my story. Not just my life compiled into chapters, but all the things I have wrestled with and discovered and overcome. The hard things as well as the good things. The extraordinary calling that I was given early in life to achieve great things, and how I came to terms with the knowledge that I would die before those things could be achieved. We all have remarkable stories. My story is no more special than anyone else's. But the legacy I want to leave is bound up in the experiences I have had, and what I have learnt through those experiences about life, love and dying.

If we had 40 more years, these are the things I would tell her myself, over time, so that Elise could draw from what I have learnt. I want her to know the peace I have known. And I want her to understand and experience the hope I have had, and the fearlessness with which I have faced not only death, but also life. But the reality is, we do not have 40 years. We have just a few more days. And in all likelihood they are days she will never recall. But Elise will have this. My story. My reflections. My heart.

———————

Dying is about the now. And there is always a new now—a new battle to be fought, a new condition to be faced. As the end approaches time does alter—your experience of it, at least. The days blur, the focus narrows, the emphasis becomes about getting through each moment. Because dying is difficult. Never let anyone say otherwise. Every day is like a mountain.

So I will begin in the now, because the now is also the end. I began these reflections four weeks ago—most of what is written in these pages was compiled over that time—and right now, as I begin, I am drawing them to a close. Signing off. Because I am tired. So tired. The fatigue that has been building over the month has been like nothing I have felt before in my life. Fatigue on a soul level, if such a thing exists. It is impossible to describe and certainly impossible to imagine. I hope you never know it.

But this is what dying is like. You can never be sure whether what you are feeling is because your organs are failing or if it is a generalised side effect of the pain medication. I am pretty sure now, though, that what I am feeling, and have been feeling over the past few weeks, is associated with the nearness of death itself. I can hear it in my voice when I speak. It is thin and dry. Making my muddled thoughts heard is a struggle. It is in the colour of my eyes when I see myself in the photos friends are taking in their goodbye moments. They are yellow and weary, and look desperate for rest.

But there is no pain. The pain is under control. At least. Just exhaustion. The exhaustion that comes when your body is giving up.

I am dying because of a complex genetic precondition called hyperplastic polyposis syndrome. It is complex because, unlike many genetic conditions, it is not just a case of something having been passed down from parents or grandparents. I *am* the family history—the first in our family to suffer this partic-ular condition, which predisposed the cells in my large intestine to suffer mutations. These mutations, in turn, resulted in uncontrolled cellular growth that my body could not, of itself, keep in check. Another way of saying this is that I got bowel cancer—cancer being, of course, the uncontrolled growth of cells that are able to evade the body's immune system. Each one of us creates cancer cells every day, but our bodies, typically, are able to recognise them and kill them before they become a problem. Occasionally, though, a cell line will be particularly aggressive and will develop the mechanism—through existing genetic machinery or through mutations—to evade the body's defences. In such cases, the cancer will thrive. If the cancer produces a tumour, it will grow until symptoms elsewhere in the body result in its discovery. We call this diagnosis. And for me, Diagnosis Day came when I was 27 years old, almost six years ago now, by which time the tumour had grown so significantly that the very best treatment available to doctors at the time—and even now—was unable to address it. And by 'address it' I mean cure it. On the day my cancer was first diagnosed, I was given a 40 per cent chance of surviving five years. I have achieved that, but only for reasons that place me outside those statistics. When they say five years, that is their way of saying 'cure'. If you live five years, chances are you will go on to live a lot longer. I am not one of those people, because the more significant diagnosis, in terms of my life expectancy, came a full year after the discovery of my cancer, when, based on the progression of the disease even after a year of chemotherapy, I was told I had around two years to live.

I have beaten that prognosis by almost three years, but now, finally, my time is up.

So here I am, propped upright in the bed I share with Hannah, in our modern, bright, two-storey suburban home in the west of Auckland, New Zealand's largest city. It is here that I will die because of the mass that is accumulating in my abdomen. The cancer is now rampant in my liver and in the tissue supplying blood to my intestines. I have partial bowel obstructions that are causing me to experience nausea, vomiting and gas, and these symptoms, in turn, are preventing me from eating. I have obstructive jaundice, which means the parts of the liver that drain bile into the gut are blocked. This condition produces its own toxic response. The body cannot survive with these blockages preventing it from doing what it needs to do. So, in about a week or so, my organs, having fought the good fight together, will fail together. Like an engine forced to run without oil or coolant, my body will experience a mechanical shutdown. It will simply grind to a halt.

When you are terminal, you think about this moment. And so you prepare for it. When you are palliative, it is almost all you think about. I moved home to die after being away from the house for eight weeks or so. I was in the hospital for a while, fighting infections and pain, and when they were brought under control I was discharged to the local hospice. In the hospice, my biggest struggle was with despondency, as I came to terms with what the end of my life actually meant. And then I was discharged to home. All of these steps were planned months ago, and come under the catch-all term 'palliative care'. And they are all being followed according to a plan called the advanced care pathway that I drew up with my doctor just a few months ago, back when I was well—so well, in fact, that it was easy to forget that I was terminal and would not see out the year. When someone tells you that your disease cannot be cured, you know this moment is coming. Some time. But I was an unusual case. I had been well for a long time before the end was apparent. And you never really know how close you are to the end. So even as I drew up my plans for dying, I never felt that death was close. Not like I do now.

How does someone die according to plan? Sure, I am dying according to my wishes and not those of anyone else. I have been fortunate that I am well enough to die at home. Many people do not have that chance. All the family are just here, and not waiting like hospital visitors for an allocated time to see me. But death is unpredictable. You can make your plans, follow your choices, make guesses about how long you have left, but the truth is, every single one of us only gets to do this once. Which means there is no rehearsal. Every experience of dying is a first time and very few of us talk about it. It is the last great taboo, and even in this moment, the very end, few people discuss what the experience is actually like. And so the fear of it accumulates.

I want to face mortality with honesty and acceptance. It is just a part of life, after all.

The process of dying has surprised me. Even as a medical doctor, I have experienced things I did not expect. And that is because experiencing dying is very different to knowing about dying. I had a rough idea what the process would be like. A month ago I could have described the types of experiences I might have, even down to when I might die. But the actual experience is something else entirely. Palliative care is described as dying made comfortable, and this is true . . . to a certain extent. But dying is neither easy nor comfortable, whatever they say. That daily mountain is soul-destroying. Physically, mentally challenging. Prolonged. Exhausting. With low moods. You feel so tired you never truly wake up.

In many ways, I am an 'ideal' candidate for palliative care at home and a relatively 'easy' death. I have my family's full support. Hannah, her mother, my parents, are around most of the time. I am a qualified doctor, which means I have some understanding of what is happening to me. And I live in a beautiful house. The windows are open most days and the earliest signs of summer are on the breeze and in the sounds of the flying insects. And yet, it has been so hard. Harder than I expected.

There have been moments when I have thought about how much easier the process of dying could be. You could just pop the required drug in an intravenous syringe and give me a quick injection, and there it is, done. I see now how, at some point, it just becomes unbearable. Of course, you cannot control when you are going to die. And that is where the whole discussion around euthanasia comes in. It is a conversation that, as a nation, we in New Zealand have not yet had. But we will eventually. They have done surveys of doctors as opposed to laypeople, ascertaining their feelings on end-of-life measures, and what they would personally opt for in order to keep themselves alive longer. And doctors invariably choose to opt out much, much sooner than laypeople. Laypeople would rather do anything they could to stay alive. A doctor says no, I have seen how people die, and that is not necessarily the right thing. I would rather die sooner.

I think I would rather die sooner than later. Our choice to go palliative was based around a decision to die rather than prolong life for as long as possible, because that would have come at the price of quality of life. Another two months of life is not so valuable if it is a miserable time. The pro-euthanasia approach to end of life advocates a specific time at which people in my position die. Invite your friends around, hold an event, book a time, and that is the end of your life. But here I am at that point, and I do not know that I agree with that approach. I have faith issues around upholding life. And as a doctor my job is to uphold life for as long as I can. But . . . I now understand why the conversation will happen, one day. Definitely.

I had laryngitis when I came home—the terminally ill still get sick, like everyone else—but I felt at peace about how my final weeks would pass. Yet despite what I know from my medical experience, and with all the support I have had, I was still unprepared for the actual challenges. Could I have been better prepared? I am not sure what I could have done differently, short of trial and error—and there is no opportunity for that. But yes, is the short answer—I could have been better prepared for dying.

What I have discovered is that dying is the great leveller. It does not matter what you know or how privileged you are, whether you have faith or whether you believe in the natural forces of the universe—or, indeed, have no faith at all. At some point in everyone's life, it comes to this. Perhaps not like this exactly. Some people die in accidents or from massive heart attacks, but many people will face death like I have. Deterioration. The gradual stripping-away of everything you are and everything you have been.

My legs were the first to go. I have an intrathecal pump that goes into my back and paralyses the pain. Like an epidural. I cannot do without it. It is because of this that I get to die at home. But in anaesthetising the pain, it pretty much paralyses my legs. The muscles in my legs are deteriorating because of lack of innervation. If you don't use it, you lose it. And so the vicious cycle goes on. Which means that for most of the past few weeks I have spent all of my time in bed. On the odd occasion I have been hoisted up so that I could spend time in the living room, but even then I was stuck in my chair, unable to move about. Bed, chair . . . at the end of the day there is not much difference. I have spent some time downstairs and have found that exhausting. I spent one morning in a recliner chair we borrowed from my parents so that I could farewell some of my closest friends from the comfort of the lounge. I was in good spirits that day, despite the emotional farewell, but the next day, then the next, and the one after . . . a gradual and noticeable decline. Thinking back over the days since then, I realise that I never recovered from the exhaustion of that goodbye.

My cognition has suffered the most. Losing mobility is difficult, but losing your capacity to think is worse. I love to imagine and to reflect. I love to write and to cogitate. All of which has been made more difficult over recent years because of chemotherapy. I have just tried to get used to that over time, and I learnt to cope with it. But coming home, those two things combined have been hard to take. I am not used to feeling confined in my own home. I love people. I love talking. I love learning and explaining complex things. But for long spells my mind has been in a fog. Alone in this room with my muddled thoughts—I was not quite ready for dying to be like this.

And yet, in spite of all this, there have been special moments. Moments when I have travelled. To places I have never been. To places on the news and places in the future. To other galaxies and other times . . .

————————

But home is where I want to die.

During the few weeks I was in the hospital, and then the hospice, there were times when I wondered whether I would ever make it home. They included some very dark days. It is difficult to come to terms with the idea that you have nothing left to fight for, particularly when you have fought for so long. To be confronted with the realisation that all you could have achieved and all you could have said are behind you . . .

But here I am, looking around me at a familiar room, with its photos of happier times, and all the things that typically belong here: the bits and pieces of a few years of marriage placed on the dresser and over on the drawers where all my medicines are stacked. I can hear familiar noises from the rooms below. I can play music on my phone. I text Hannah and she brings my pain relief. Mum is here most days too, and she brings food, or coffee, or cleans me up after a vomit.

In some ways, being home is a bittersweet experience. You are reminded daily of the things you would rather be doing around the place. Everything but sitting here. Mowing the lawns and smelling the garden, for example. Or cooking. Being in this place where I have enjoyed so many good times over recent months reminds me that those times are over. It brings to mind all the things I can no longer do. And the things that have not yet been done.

I am not despondent about this, though. Home is where I want to be. Because home is where Hannah is. And home is where Elise is.

She comes to sit on the bed for her playtime with Daddy. Despite the full beard I have grown and the glasses I wear now because my eyes are too dry for contact lenses, her eyes light up when she sees me. She grew so much in the first eight months of her life. And she was spoilt, too, what with two stay-at-home parents for almost all of that time. She changed so much while I was in the hospital, and then in the hospice. This was its own marker of time. So much development that I missed in such a short period. I look at Elise sometimes and see a different baby—each day something new. New skills she learns. Fine motor control she is developing so quickly. New things she is able to do. Milestones she is reaching all the time. We watch for them, Hannah and I, as doctors more so than parents, those subtle signs of development that other parents might miss.

In all of these things, I have had to come to terms with letting go. When I cry with Hannah, in the evenings when we are finally alone, it is because of what I will miss out on in years to come. In a strange way this is what gives me peace. The knowledge that there is little point prolonging my life as I currently have it helps me to welcome my own mortality. It is not another playtime on the bed that I want. It is a lifetime. I want to be there for Elise's first day of school, and for her first friendships, boys, learning new things, discovering the world, broadening her understanding of other people and of the privilege she was born into.

I can hear Elise shouting for attention downstairs. Hannah will be preparing her lunch while Elise's grandmother helps out—with the laundry perhaps, or by taking her for a long walk when lunch is done. On the fridge door our names are linked together in oversized Scrabble tiles, and when the door is open you can see these names as you approach the house from the long driveway. Hannah and I have talked about the future, and these have been some of the hardest conversations for me. But even in this I have found peace, even in accepting there will be a time when my name is no longer on the fridge door.

Elise will not remember this time. And for Hannah, this period will be a blip one day. In 30 years, these six years will be a distant memory. I hope they will be a significant memory, and that the memory shapes Hannah for all of that time, but she will move on. That is what I hope, anyway. I want Hannah to follow her own dreams. And who knows? Perhaps they will include the vision we discussed beside a fireplace one cold Australian morning several years ago, when it became clear to both of us that we had discovered someone with whom we could spend the rest of our lives.

———

This has been the stuff of my reflections in these last weeks—the people, the places, the goals and purposes, and also the things I have had to let go. It has been a time of submission, to a degree, of coming to terms with questions and unresolved issues that I have, in faith, hoped to find answers for but have conceded when those answers have not come. It is not true that all things are resolved on the eve of dying. There are loose threads and story arcs that have not reached their conclusions. It is in submission to an unseen, bigger picture, that I have been able to find peace, if not resolution.

The word 'uncertainty' has come to me a lot in this final stage. It best describes how I felt when I came home to face the final weeks. Uncertainty. It fits how I feel spiritually, too, as I ponder the absence of assurances I might have expected. Uncertainty. Even so, for me, this was never scary like it is for many. Perhaps that is because I have accepted the outcome. I know it is not like this for everyone. Some people fight to stay alive for as long as they can, and never give up on the belief that somehow their struggle will stave off death. It never does, though. It merely fills their final days with pain and suffering on a deeply emotional level.

I gave up fighting some time ago. What I battle now is the growing heaviness that dying imposes on me in other ways— the daily struggle to not suffer too much. Four weeks ago, my suspicion, both as a doctor and as the patient, was that I would survive another five to six weeks. That is almost upon me, and my estimate is proving accurate. I felt after the first week that dying would have its own 'normal' state. By that, I mean the approach of death would bring its own symptoms. And that also has been true. You can never know, of course, whether what you are feeling is a temporary or permanent state, but in my case, the deep fatigue and general feeling of unwellness that I began to feel early did, in fact, become the new normal.

So, while I speak of weeks, and days, and know that today is September 24 because I have seen the date on my phone, the days of the week have no meaning to me. Monday or Saturday, whether it is the weekend or not the weekend—it means little. Such markers of time are for the living, not the dying. Passages of time are marked by the visits of friends, or dinnertime, or my evenings with Hannah. I watch the news now and then. Even this close to the end I am interested in current events. The New Zealand election. The rise of Islamic State. The announcement of the latest iPhone. A free album from U2. But, for the most part, time passes me by. I have become insignificant to time, and soon it will run me over. I wear a watch on my wrist but have no need to check it. Indeed, it hangs so loosely off my skinny arm that it best serves to remind me how much weight I have lost in such a short period. The watch was given to me by Mum and Dad as a combined birthday and graduation gift in 2011. I wrote at the time that my watches tend to last about eight years, so I need to make sure it is one I love to look at every day. But I knew then, as I do now for certain, that the watch would outlast me.

Where is God in this? I have been asked this question many times. It is a good and fair question, particularly for someone of faith. And the answer is not obvious. I have been around faith and questions of faith my whole life. I was raised in an evangelical faith tradition, among a faith community, and with a faith that I came to call my own. But my journey has not been typical, and the issues I have had to wrestle with during my illness have brought me to conclusions that have been out of step with many people in that faith tradition. I have always been honest about my questions and doubts as much as I have my beliefs. And even now, when you might expect God to be closer than ever, my actual experience has been otherwise. In my faith tradition, people typically speak of triumphing over adversity, or of the good things that God brings about when a righteous person suffers. I think they believe such pithy sayings will ease the burden of what you are experiencing. But long before I was diagnosed with cancer, I knew that the issues around why we suffer and where we find hope are more complex than typical Christian platitudes allow. My experiences over the past few years have confirmed my suspicions. Nevertheless, without the faith that has been sharply honed in my own experience of suffering, I would not have known the peace that has accompanied me through this whole time. I have discovered things about meaning and purpose and love and community that may never have occurred to me in different circumstances.

In the final third of my life, I was driven by a sense of calling that emerged from this faith, and which gave purpose to my whole concept of what life could be. I had the conviction of a bigger vision that my sickness has actively destroyed. For me, suffering has been no passive thing I have had to endure, but an actual destructive force that has altered the course of my life and prevented those things from being achieved. So convinced am I of my calling that were I healed tomorrow, it would still be the thing that drove me.

I say this knowing that I am not likely to be healed. I have asked for it, certainly. Many times, in fact. Hannah and I, both of us, have asked God to step in and do something miraculous. And why not?

Immediately after Diagnosis Day, I saw my sickness as a hurdle. I never thought it would mean the end of a vision. But healing did not come. And then I was terminal. I suppose that in my mind I always expected I would be one of the 40 per cent who make it. But with my terminal diagnosis came the recognition that the vision I had been given was unlikely ever to be realised. Either that, or something miraculous was going to happen to make it possible. And along the way, that miracle appeared to be a possibility—just a possibility, but a big one. My mind has gone back to that time repeatedly over recent weeks. Interesting that, as the end looms larger, my mind goes back to the hope that might have been.

There is an Old Testament character, Job, whose claim to fame is the suffering he endured, for no apparent reason, and how he refused to curse God in the midst of it. His friends come to him with all the theological reasons they can muster for why he is suffering, none of which make sense to Job, who becomes even more miserable the more they speak. I have no more answers than old Job, but like him I can say I have never genuinely been angry with God. Not even now. I have been tearful, to be sure. And those tears have increased. But the answers to my questions . . . in some ways they got waylaid while I fought the more important battle of staying alive. But now? Still no answers. Am I at peace with the lack of resolution? Have I fully let go? Is there a part of me that wants to understand the biggest question of my life in the short time I have left?

Perhaps my questions have been replaced with hope. Because I still do have hope. Hope that I can die soon and that my suffering will be over. Hope that the moments I have remaining are meaningful for Hannah. Hope that I can leave Elise with something significant, memorable, a glimpse of me. Hope that God is loving and is, indeed, journeying with me even now, through my suffering.

The very presence of love in this house, through the care and attention of my wife, and my parents, and Hannah's parents, my siblings and friends, has made me think of God's presence in a new way. And yet . . . I still wonder whether there is more that I could feel . . . more that God could give me.

―――――――

In the absence of that 'more', though, I have the moment. I have learnt to value the moment above all else, no matter what the moment consists of. This, in itself, is an act of faith—to trust the present.

We take so much for granted while we live with no thought of dying, but for so long now dying has been part of my everyday reality. I have discovered that suffering puts our fears, hopes, desires and dreams into a bigger context. To know that you will die helps you recognise how trivial are the things you allow to dominate your time and emotions. In the face of so much that we take too seriously, I have learnt to be thankful that I am alive, I am breathing in the fresh air, I am waking up in the morning, I am enjoying a roof over my head.

I have a handful of moments left. That is all. But that is everything. It is in the moment that I can stave off the effects of the dying haze and reflect just a little more on what remains . . . the meaning, significance and purpose of these last days. Because every moment matters, and I can appreciate the now until there is no now left. And who knows? Perhaps there will be something I say in that moment that brings me to life in her mind and helps Elise remember. Because that is my greatest hope. To give her just a glimpse of who I was. Of who I am.

And then I will die.

CHAPTER 2
Every moment counts

All of a sudden, every moment counts, be it the ordinary or the extraordinary, the mundane or the special. I get frustrated that my cerebrum, doing what it is supposed to do, is stealing my moments from me. I don't want my life to disappear into an abyss of faint memories, I want it to be real, I want it to be present, I want it to be experiential.

I'm training myself to change this . . . if that is at all possible.

Life is far too valuable to let skip by.

'Every moment', The Boredom Blog, November 21, 2009

The beginning of the story, for me, is no more than flashes of memory, images of landscapes and streets, rooms in houses, grandparents saying goodbye in the driveway of a suburban house. I remember schools, the faces of children, particular feelings associated with different settings. My early years were spent here, there and everywhere, which carved more memories in my mind of my childhood experiences than other people typically have of theirs. We moved around so much that my various memory flashes are attached to different houses, particular landmarks. From my very earliest days I had a sense of stories and people and episodes from my life being placed against actual settings: the convergence of time and space and how stories emerge from the simultaneous existence of multiple elements—characters, places, so-called coincidences, unique moments that go towards assembling an entire life, a unique life, lived in a way that no one at any other time has ever lived theirs. And a story that, when you are dead, is gone for good.

But I was born in a very unremarkable manner, in the middle of nowhere, in a small town in New Zealand's central North Island, back in the days of three-digit phone numbers and a telephone exchange manned by an actual human being. My dad was a mechanic in the early days, but his drive to improve his career took us around the country for my entire childhood. I learnt early that 'home', as a concept, was not about a town, or a house, or a district—it was about family. I have wanted to travel my whole life, and I am certain that it was during these years that the bug took hold.

But these snippets of memory I have been recalling at random in recent days . . . flashing images of snow, would you believe? Nothing significant, but a clear memory of grandparents visiting and all of us going outside to build a snowman. But we also have photos of that, so who can say whether it is my actual memory or a fictional memory I have built up around the pictures. I do remember school, though. Very vague memories of my first school days, right at the end of the school year because I was desperate to begin. We were in the city by then, while Dad was studying to be a teacher, and the end of his studies coincided with me turning five, finally old enough to begin. So I remember the school, and my first school days, literally weeks before the end of the summer break, and the house we lived in at the time. I remember the birth of my sister, and the move to Rotorua at the end of the year. And I remember three different houses in Rotorua, three different primary schools, some of the kids—vague, nondescript memories, but a clear impression of change, and adaptation, and movement. I remember, too, a lifestyle block where we lived and where Dad could revive his own memories of growing up on a dairy farm. We had sheep and cows, a goat, land to run around.

And I remember, too, that it was about the time Halley's Comet came whipping through. We went over to a friend's house because he had a telescope, and everyone took turns at having a look at the comet. I remember that as I looked through the telescope at the night sky and the millions of stars, and gained my first real impression of the vast expanse of space, I had no clue what I was looking at. I remember hearing voices that said, 'Did you see it, did you see it?' And I said yes. But I had no idea. Everyone else saw it. Or at least they said they saw it. Just not me.

One of my life's regrets actually, not seeing Halley's Comet. I wish I had been older. I would quite like to have seen it.

One day, perhaps.

———

As I look back over my life, and particularly these past few years, from the standpoint of this time and place and the simultaneous existence of everything that has converged to make me who I am in the story of this moment—this bed, this room, my condition, the people who surround me—I can see what I would describe as a divine thread: the convergence of time lines, sequences of events, certain people, doors that were opened, opportunities that suggest the hand of God. I say this as a person with a Christian faith. Someone who does not share this perspective could easily call it all coincidence, or the work of the universe, or random occurrences—each of them different types of faith, I suppose. And I admit that anyone reflecting on their life as I have done in recent weeks is prone to crafting a narrative that makes sense of where they have been and where they have arrived, perhaps even assigning value to things that had none at the time. I also know that in the moment, in the context of these events, I did not necessarily recognise a divine influence as I claim to now.

It is not uncommon for people approaching death to contemplate spiritual matters for the first time. Death has a way of bringing many things into focus, including latent beliefs in God and questions about what happens beyond death—if there is anything beyond death at all. For me, though, such thoughts have always been there. If anything, I am actually contemplating such things less now than I did in the past. Faith has shaped my life and who I am from an early age. And when I talk about seeing a divine thread, I am not just talking about the past six years of sickness—it goes back further, back before med school, before my first degree, even into high school. In fact, my first awakenings to how faith was influencing the way I saw such things as inequality and lack of privilege were happening in my intermediate school years, around the ages of eleven and twelve.

The classic Christian story of how one man's extreme suffering somehow represented the divine love for humanity was one in which I was happy to locate my own understanding of myself, and also how I understood the workings of a world where such persecution was possible. If Jesus was God, then the fact that we took him and brutally tortured him said a lot to me about humanity's capacity for great cruelty and stupidity.

I did not think these things as a little kid, of course. They came later. But what I did notice in my very first school years were the students who had nothing, who went to school in bare feet, who never seemed to have lunch. From around the age of five I was beginning to recognise certain things about my world. The first was the Maori culture into which I had been placed. It was as normal to me as a European culture is to kids in the city. I noticed some of the poverty that was attached to that culture, too, but that never seemed to diminish its richness. I was aware also that my family was Christian, that church and a faith community were as natural for us as family dinners.

Faith was always going to play a major role in my story, for the simple fact that it was such an integral part of my family life. But it was not the only factor that would shape who I am and the direction my life would take. Sure, church life was ever present in my childhood. Our family was Baptist and my dad pursued theological studies during my early childhood years, before taking up pastoral and teaching roles in different places in the North Island. So, for me, faith was interwoven with my growing sense that home was not about a fixed place, but about relationships. At the same time, my exposure to Maori education and culture was solidifying in me the presence in this world of other values, other ideas and different levels of privilege. An awareness of others, and of otherness itself, was a core value from an early age.

This was underscored in later years when we returned to the city and I attended a school in one of the wealthier inner-city suburbs. I went from running around at lunchtime in bare feet to running around with kids who wore Nike Air Jordans and Reebok Pumps. What is more, if their shoes broke they would have a brand-new pair the very next day. I had never known anything like this, this amount of affluence. Coming from a family where Dad was pursuing ongoing studies, we fell on the lower end of the scale in terms of wealth. This was a whole different league to what I had seen anywhere. It was also a very sudden exposure to an Asian culture as opposed to a Maori one. I had never been to a school populated by Asians before, let alone Asians who were so wealthy. It shaped my world view enormously. Even as a kid I saw the divide between those with and those without, but this did not make me feel underprivileged. The opposite, in fact. It made me feel special. My value was not in the sneakers I could afford to wear, but in my ability to recognise difference.

I was also becoming aware of what I wanted to be. Or, at least, becoming aware of which disciplines or fields of knowledge I wanted to pursue. If you had asked me at the age of eight or nine what I wanted to be when I grew up, my answers would have been typical of any kid that age—I would have said a fireman or a policeman. Before long, though, I was recognising that science had always intrigued me. And I had an inquisitive mind. The birthday presents that stand out in my memory are the electronic build sets my parents would buy.

And all this was emerging as faith was becoming my own. When you grow up in a family of faith you can go along for years without that faith being yours—without really understanding yourself in light of that faith story. You can describe yourself as a Christian, and perhaps, as I had, you can even have said the prayer asking to be 'saved', but what that all means does not necessarily occur to you—happy though you are to be part of it all. In my case, I would not claim the faith until the age of fifteen, when I made the decision to be baptised. There was a fundamental shift at this point. Faith was no longer just the family tradition, or the doctrine of the church community to which I belonged and the practices I followed because I always had. It was about knowledge, essentially, and about consciously acknowledging that the story of faith is one that influenced my own ways of understanding and engaging with life. It is a wilful act of submission to a historical story about Jesus and who he claimed to be, and to the confessions of the community of faith that sprang up around him—particularly concerning the events associated with his death and resurrection, the Easter story. For me, this was why it was impossible to separate faith from the issues of life and death—they are part of the same story. There is no Christian faith, not even a Christian story, without those elements of the human drama with which we spend most of our life engaging—life, death, love, hope. When I recognised this, and grasped this story as my own, my life took a very specific path. I knew that my own life would also engage with the human drama and its fundamental questions. I did not necessarily know how.

So faith, to me, went hand in hand with an inner rage I felt about injustice. That manifested itself in the way I noticed even in school how some kids seemed to have so much when others had so little, through to recognising how corporations and governments could cause and sustain the suffering of entire peoples in underdeveloped and impoverished nations. When I say 'rage', I am not talking about anger or a desire to cause violence. I borrow the word from the band Rage Against the Machine, who were big when my musical tastes were forming in my teens. Their lyrics against injustice and exploitation were as formative to my faith as biblical verses. This 'rage', which in some ways is synonymous with my faith, energised my travels, my studies, my desire to do medicine, and, in the years I have been sick, my hope that my own suffering, and what I have discovered about life in the midst of it, would help others who were confronted with similar challenges.

I have been thinking of Matt and Cara, my brother and sister, as I reflect on my early years. How could I not? We were all born into the same family of faith, and faith has influenced all our lives and still does. They have watched my deterioration in recent weeks, as have friends and family, and while they do not say anything to me, I know they are finding this difficult.

They are both younger than me, and the genetic nature of my illness has changed their lives—five-yearly checks for them to ensure they do not follow the medical trajectory I have now established. Behind me on the wall is a painting from my sister. She is the arty one, the educator and the innovator. My brother is into numbers and decimal points. I got on better with him than her as children, but after leaving home I realised it was because she and I were so similar. By that I mean we are both stubborn. He is an introvert, like Hannah, and my sister is extroverted like me. I am not an artist like her, though—not by any stretch of the imagination.

I see them once or twice a week, and I am always conscious of the changes they are seeing in me from week to week. I deteriorate so much on a daily basis, in terms of my colour, my energy, the weakness in my voice, that to see me after a break of only a handful of days must come as a bit of a shock.

But they keep it to themselves.

———

Back when I had the time to write—back before I succumbed to the joys of being a stay-at-home dad who could suspend reality and convince himself he was not sick at all—I planned to take all the themes associated with faith from the blog I have written for six years and explore them in greater depth. I did not have the answers to those issues, necessarily, but I knew they warranted further thought. I have found that issues of faith are more than questions of spirituality. They are the stuff of life and death, meaning and purpose, joy and sorrow—the elements of the human drama.

But my final bout of sickness came upon me suddenly, disrupting the idyllic lifestyle Hannah and I had established for ourselves and our small family over this past year. And I missed my chance. So here they are instead at the beginning of these final reflections—an appropriate place, I think, considering faith has been interwoven with my story from its beginning to the very end.

My sense of God over these past few weeks at home has not been what I expected. At this moment, feeling as I do, I would say that I am slowly welcoming him. And by that I mean I am preparing myself to die. I do not necessarily feel that God is close, or that I am about to die. But I am ready. Ready in a way that I was not ready four weeks ago, or even two weeks ago. I am ready to be embraced. And that is a comforting feeling.

There is no distress in this for me. The only distress I am feeling is physical, the constant and mounting fatigue. Spiritually, I am completely at peace with where I am and where I am going. And even in that, I have very few thoughts about what comes next. I believe there is life after death, in spite of my medical training and the scientific methodologies in which I have been schooled—and with which, I should add, I am very comfortable. But while I believe there is something more—a resurrection life, so to speak—it is a mystery to me, and I am happy for it to remain so. I will discover what it is when I get there.

But regarding the question of God's presence, which I have pondered on and off during this whole palliative phase, I have to be honest: I have not felt God as I might have expected, or certainly as I hoped. And when I use the term 'God's presence' I am remembering moments in years past, when there was an emotional element to my faith experience, on particular occasions and with certain people, that I associated with God being close. That is what I have hoped for in this last phase of the faith journey. At the beginning of this time at home I would have said I hoped for it more than anything. I knew then that it was a juvenile hope, a regression to a less mature faith, even. Over the years, and with getting older and more 'mature' in my faith, I have moved away from emotion-based faith experiences, but what has surprised me over recent weeks is that it has often been what I wanted most.

I have blamed myself for its absence. I have blamed my own lack of discipline in working as I have in the past at putting myself in the space to know the presence of God. In my experience of faith, the returns have come with the more effort I have put in. It is the same as any investment you make—you take a risk and hopefully see a return, and the greater the risk the bigger the reward. To some degree my life has been this way. There have been opportunities to step out in faith and they have generally resulted in the experience of a fuller life. Love may be totally synonymous with God's character, but if you do not want it you will not see it. The flip side of this is that you can be in a place of absolute despair, utterly bereft, but if you reach out for it that love is right there, at any point in life. That is what I have discovered, anyway. Even now, I am not feeling utterly bereft. I have been there before so I know what it is like. And yet, have I reached out to grasp that experience I know is just around the corner? Perhaps not.

I have wondered at times over recent weeks whether I could have done more to feel that love. By 'more' I mean the typical devotional disciplines—reading the Bible, prayer, contemplation. But the truth is, I have been too tired and too muddled in the head to give them more time or energy. Someone suggested to me that a loving God would not wait for a dying man to work harder before showing up. Perhaps that is true. Even for me there have been moments when I have allowed myself to say, 'God . . . where are you?'

But as the days have progressed, I have recognised more and more that God's presence is here in a way I had not counted on—through the nearness of people, and through their service and their attention and their care. I have come to see more vividly the importance of a community of people who have travelled with me through the broken landscape of my sickness, and through them I have come to see more the importance of community—not just to my faith, but to my humanity. I have come to see God's love from a wholly new perspective. There is a prevailing idea in my faith tradition that suffering is meaningful because it makes us turn to God. This is a problematic idea, because it sometimes results in people believing that suffering is a prerequisite to knowing God. But I think there is a component of truth in the idea that when we suffer we tend to turn to God more. That is not just my experience, but the experience of poets and hymn writers and church leaders who have said the same for more than 2000 years. The hymn 'Amazing Grace' would not have been written were it not for this reality. But it is not the whole truth—not by any means. I do not believe that suffering is a requirement for knowing God, but I believe that love is.

And where love is concerned, my dying has allowed me to experience what I have come to describe as the great reversal. Here I am, lying in bed, incapable of doing most of the things for myself that I need just to make it through the day, let alone to the end. It has been a humbling thing, to come home so that my wife can nurse me, and so that my family and faith community can support me. I never saw my life going this way. I was meant to be the giver, not the receiver, of this type of love. And accepting this, and then receiving it—and receiving it not just as the charity of other people, but as the very loving presence of God—has been one of my biggest personal challenges.

I have come to a place of acceptance in these things . . . and so I continue to trust. And in trusting, I feel peace in the moment. From the beginning of this process, to now, there has never been a point when I have not trusted or when I have even questioned whether that trust was legitimate. When I think of the things that have got me through, trust has been at the heart. On diagnosis, then around the relapses that took away what little hope we were given along the way, I have been faced with the need to trust. I came to see that trusting in God was like being presented with a series of doors. Life offers us all kinds of doors, leading to all kinds of outcomes, and we can spend so much futile time trying every single door, for escape, or meaning, or relief, or significance—whatever it is we feel we need. But we avoid the door that requires us to trust whatever it is we trust in. For me, as a person of faith, that is God. And from Diagnosis Day, I have walked through that last door first. Why? Because I had nothing else. Which other door could I choose? I knew immediately that I could not rely on myself to change anything about what I was facing—not my strength, not my character, not my learning. All I had was this prayer: 'The only way I am going to get through this is by trusting you.'

I remember a night alone in hospital, a week after my initial surgery. The histology had come back confirming the tumour was cancer. It was a brief moment of emotional turmoil. I was reading the Bible on my phone and ended up saying to myself, 'What can you do when you come to a place such as this, when you have just been told you have cancer?' That was the moment when I knew the only door available to me was the last one. Would I have taken other doors if they were presented as genuine options? Maybe. But I had no options. And as soon as I trusted, I felt a release. I felt peace. Trust and peace sit side by side, because once you have chosen to go through the last door, the futility of trying all the other doors ends. And once you experience peace, you know that it was the right door to take all along.

From that moment, my understanding and expression of faith changed. I think you experience trust at a deeper level once you have handed yourself over to it. My life had prepared me for this decision. I am sure it is not so easy to trust when you never have before. And I know that some people die of a terminal illness without ever trusting. They fight to the end. But I had been readied for this by a lifetime of faith, for which I have been thankful every day of the past six years.

Had I not had that . . . I cannot bear to contemplate the alternative. To be in this place now and not be at peace, or to have faced the toughest challenges of recent years without trust? I would not have it any other way.

Sometimes life brings us so low that the only thing left is to trust in God. I know that for many people that is nonsense, and as a man of science I understand that response. But in my story, the peace I have experienced throughout this journey has been a happy outcome of being shown the last door first, and walking through it knowing it was the only option I had.

If I were to summarise my faith in simple terms, I would say that since I decided to be baptised I have had a deep sense that something bigger is going on that I do not necessarily understand but am a part of. This macro view of faith has helped me integrate the things I believe with science, which is fundamentally distinct from theology. When I left school I did a Bachelor of Science degree but also completed an Introduction to Theology paper at a local theological college. I wanted to bring the two disciplines together, at least in my own mind. In my understanding, they had no need to be so independent from one another.

For as long as I can remember, the way I think has been analytical and process-driven. For some people this results in a cynical view of anything that cannot be demonstrated scientifically, but I have always known that there is something spiritual going on, something bigger that cannot be quantified by science. With faith, I had a reassurance that if my scientific foundations were to fall down, my belief set would not. It was not a backup plan so much as a foundation. Not that I held one set of foundational beliefs over the other. I have always tried to integrate faith with the day-to-day realities of my life—science, economics, medicine, politics.

My decision to be baptised came after an intense period of unhappiness at school. Another move out of the city in my teens saw us relocate to Hawkes Bay, to the east of the North Island, a brand-new experience in terms of culture, values and environment. It was the hardest period of my pre-adult life, a time of difficult adjustments, isolation and loneliness, and a sense of being somewhat adrift. I was plundering the New Testament to get a grounding in foundational stories of faith, probably in an attempt to find stability at a time when life was not giving me any. I remember a youth camp during this period, and the discovery that there were many other teenagers who, just like me, were attempting to reconcile faith with school and family life and all they entailed. It was there that I had one of those experiences I have yearned for in recent days: a tangible feeling that God was present and was actually speaking to me—not audibly, but just about. It was so clear. What I heard was that it was time to be baptised—in other words, time to let these foundational faith stories become my own, and allow my life to be given direction and shape by them. It was transformational. It was no longer just my family's faith, it was *my* faith.

I changed from that moment—my thinking, my behaviour, and ultimately my dreams and goals. Other people noticed the changes, too. But I would not hear from God again in quite the same way until it was time to steer my professional life in a wholly new direction.

One of the earliest indications of this new direction came during my tertiary science studies. As I think over those years now, the actual degree has faded into the past, but standing out from that time is a three-week trip to the Philippines I undertook with a youth group I was in at the time. It was a short-term mission trip, and I was so passionate about it that I raised funds to enable me to go. It was consistent with the hunger that was already building in me to travel and see how people live differently in other parts of the world. It was how I first defined this feeling as a calling, a calling to overseas work in some form. And that calling is as strong today as it always was, no matter how close I am to death.

In the lead-up to the trip, I heard several people preaching or teaching about their time in overseas mission work, and I remember being captivated by the question of how I could live with greater purpose and meaning than I currently was. The trip itself opened up my eyes and heart. So much of the world lives in abject poverty—how could I justify living in the first world without guilt when so much suffering was going on? I knew I would not be able to sit idly by while the scales were so unbalanced.

That I had this awakening during my Bachelor of Science presented a problem. How were my studies consistent with a calling to overseas work? I was two years into the degree and trying to integrate my academic work with this new passion. It was in this context that I applied for med school for the second time. I had already tried once before, at the end of high school, and failed. I failed the second time as well. In the years between then and now I have reconciled those failed attempts with an appreciation, in faith and in hindsight, for a bigger story that was going on for me. The timing was not right. There was no prompting from God, for example—no sense that I was being called into medicine. I applied the first time because I was smart enough. I applied the second time because to me medicine would be the perfect vehicle by which I would get overseas, but I submitted neither application with any great conviction.

And so I took a different path.

———————————

My ongoing connection to the community in which my faith has been grounded in recent years takes place every Sunday evening, when several members of that community gather around my bed to talk, pray and say goodbye. The community exists in parallel with the café we own as a collective and through which we try to build a larger community in a defined area clustered around it, beside the railway lines running west out of the city. In some ways the story of my cancer is synonymous with the story of the community. It was forming just as I was diagnosed, and in some senses its story has been the same honest wrestle with suffering and hope, love and healing that I have been engaged in. The reality of my illness, and particularly my terminal diagnosis, has been a personal and living reminder to this community that faith is never practised in isolation from our human struggles. Faith exists right in the midst of our struggles and is never purely academic or theoretical. The questions people of faith have about God and God's involvement in the human drama are the same questions a young man dying of cancer asks every day and that help him bear up under the weight of the cruel ironies of his life.

Each Sunday, I see the impact of my dying on the faces of my friends, the people who have been closest to me outside of my immediate family throughout this journey, and who have walked beside me. They were here three nights ago, perhaps for the last time. It is up to me whether or not they come again before I am gone, but that will depend on how I feel four days from now.

There were tears on Sunday. There are not always tears. But on Sunday the group turned up all chipper, and as always asked me how I was. When I told them, it was like the air had been sucked from the room. It turns out telling your friends that you will probably be dead within the fortnight is something of a downer. Not that they needed me to tell them. Just like my brother and sister, they can see the decline. And, like them, they keep it to themselves.

But this is what being in a community is all about. You get to travel with one another through the ragged wastelands as well as the meadows. This particular community of faith is not a church, as such—it is a small group of believers who embrace the concept 'We *are* the church, we don't *go* to church' and in so doing seek to create community and be a positive influence in their neighbourhood. In our case, that neighbourhood is urban, transient, young, professional, academic. Back before its formation, I found myself in churches that fit a certain model for the sake of it, because that is what churches have always done. Encouraged by like-minded people, I yearned for a faith community that existed to enable its members to make a difference in the world, to build community out there in powerful ways. I realised that so many functions of the traditional church only make sense within the paradigm of that very tradition. They seem to serve no greater purpose on behalf of humanity, whether in the community around them or overseas in completely different cultures. There is a reason people in their young adult years are leaving churches in record numbers. Traditional forms of faith are not addressing the issues that are most pressing in society and that demand some seriously sophisticated thought and tough engagement. A radical rethink was required. But then again, loose practices become traditions over time because elements of them truly work and are relevant no matter what the surrounding society is up to. No model is perfect. I was not so radical as to think the baby should be thrown out with the bath water.

And so, six years ago, I was among a small group to start this faith community, meeting regularly to explore how to live and be part of the wider community of people who live and work hereabouts and may not even profess any faith. The community began as my own life was undergoing some fundamental changes. First, I was newly married to Hannah, and our first home was the very flat in which the fledgling community was meeting. It was the hub of the community outreach that would eventually emanate from that building on a daily basis. We lived there because it was vacant and because it was convenient. Had we not, our involvement in the community might never have happened.

But then I got sick, and from that moment our story and the story of the group became entwined. The truth is, Hannah and I were headed away from the city, probably for good. Just a week before Diagnosis Day, our friends held a farewell event for us. I like to stir by claiming, 'If you try to leave, you get cancer,' but so far this rule has only applied to me. Our plans would have taken us in a very different direction to that of the friends who weekly come to visit me now. But that is how life goes sometimes. We are still bound together, still journeying together, and they are still the ones who remain with me to the end, shedding tears because of the deterioration they see happening to me.

What does the death of someone in so tight a community mean to that group? It is hard for me to contemplate as the one who is leaving. It is something the group itself will reflect on in its own way and in its own time. But with any close-knit group, the loss of just one person can feel like the snagging of a thread in a tapestry. I think it will continue to challenge their beliefs about who God is and how God operates. I have tried to live in a way that does not shy away from asking the hard questions and openly debating the answers. I have wanted my death to be an exercise that builds their faith, not one that destroys it. I have seen how the deaths of many young people become a faith-destroying process for the families left behind. They have expectations of God, about how God should act in such a situation. Perhaps they also have notions of justice or fairness, or certain beliefs about healing. There is a prevailing view that faith should be rewarded, that it follow a cause and effect or blessing and curse formula. God's response is prescribed for him—or so they believe. And when things do not play out the way they expect, 'faith' is abandoned.

I have been very open with my community about my journey with cancer and faith, but just because we have faced these questions together does not mean we have all come to the same conclusions. Like any community, my faith community is a living organism, a dynamic group of individuals who have their own struggles, however they engage with mine. Some have their own health issues, and what has become very apparent is that just because I think a certain way about suffering and dying and God's part in that, not everybody does. As to why I think the way I do and have accepted things the way I have when others have found it very difficult to do so . . . I do not know. But I am glad that they think for themselves, and I am happy that there is no automatic acceptance of the conclusions I have reached. We all suffer in our own way. We all experience faith in our own way. And we all die in our own way. Every one of us has to say goodbye to our community, or to our family, or to our friends, in our own way—and in our own time.

That said, farewelling some friends is harder than others.

I never really accounted for the fact that I had to farewell people. In all my thinking, and in the planning I have done for these last days, I never considered what saying goodbye would be, or even whether or not it would happen. To be honest, I figured I would just see them, then one day I would stop seeing them. This has not turned out to be the case. I have said farewell to different people in their own ways, each goodbye emotional, each one exhausting.

I said farewell to my closest friend a little more than a week ago. I spent the morning downstairs in the recliner rocker and for the first time in days I had some energy. Only days before I had been desperate for the fatigue to stop and for the end to come, wondering why on earth my body was still holding on.

I knew this farewell was coming. His overseas trip had been planned for months and I knew that farewelling him would coincide with the start of his trip. So there were tears. Of course there were. We have been friends since before the formation of the group, since before marriage, before medicine. He has been there at some of the key moments in my journey over the past ten or so years.

How do you farewell someone you know so well? When you are men of faith, and also such good friends, you do not really say farewell. You say, 'See you on the other side.'

The journey of faith is almost done for me. As I said at the start, I am slowly welcoming God—welcoming a God who has always welcomed me.

I have said things to God along the way. Asked for things, too—things like healing. Mainly I have asked for peace and comfort, and for stamina. There have been truly miserable times, and it is common to fear those, so, I have asked for the courage to get through. And I am almost through.

And the healing? I have never asked for healing the way a child might ask Father Christmas for an expensive toy. I have asked for healing if it is possible in the context of the bigger story—the one I believe in but do not necessarily understand. And healing has not come.

I have never despaired because of this, though. Faith is a framework through which we engage with realities, not with fairy tales or illusions. My own story, in which I have not experienced miraculous healing, sets me apart from many of the triumphant stories that are often peddled as proof that faith works or God is real. The message about how well your life will go if you are a Christian is largely nonsense. The people peddling it are selling false hope. Church services are replete with stories about good things happening to people who pray for them. The alternative stories are rarely told, because who wants to hear from someone who has experienced suffering and loss? There is a selection bias in the public-relations mechanism surrounding faith, which means the people who did not get healed are rarely heard. Because they died.

But in my case, my faith community got to hear from someone who did not get healed. They got to hear from the guy who died. It is one of the things I hope for as I die—that I challenged people of faith to be pragmatic and to deal with realities, not with illusion.

I followed a pretty decent blueprint in this approach to faith and suffering. Jesus himself, facing death by torture the very next day, kneels in a garden, full of anxiety, and asks God to come up with a different plan. He wants a plan that does not include the suffering that is about to take place. But then, in the very next breath, he says that if there is no other way, he will submit to what is coming.

My life of faith for six years has been about living that prayer—asking for a way out but submitting to whatever comes if there is no alternative way, and asking for the strength to do so. It was only by faith that I could accept my circumstances without getting angry and without being frustrated, but the two parts of that equation have coexisted daily. They do so even now. Here, at the end, I still find myself asking for a way out. And if there is no way, for help to follow the path I am on with courage, peace and grace.

As a doctor, I have seen many people receive bad news. They have come to mind over the past weeks, for obvious reasons. I have seen a full spectrum of responses, depending on the particular person's beliefs, philosophies and ideas. For many people, the easiest and most comfortable response is denial. Some are angry and look for someone or something to blame, while others keep their reactions to themselves, so that you cannot tell how they are processing the news. But you can pick the ones who go into denial, because the things they say in response to their diagnosis do not acknowledge its magnitude.

I never had the luxury of denial. My training made certain of that. I understood my situation pretty well, right from the start. With that particular coping mechanism withheld from me, what could I do but confront the realities and bring my faith to bear upon them?

The upshot of all this? It is very simple: every moment counts. When you are not wasting time and energy on denial; and when you are not getting angry because your expectations of God or the universe or your spouse have not been met; and when you are not filled with fear about what is to come, or regret about what you have left behind . . . right there is the moment. And moments filled with life and grace and wonder, not to mention peace and hope and courage, are moments worth cherishing.

During my illness, such moments have been magnified in my appreciation. I once wrote about noticing the colours of autumn in a whole new way because I did not know if I would ever experience autumn again. Christmas Day. Birthdays. Graduation. My first day at work. Moments that were suddenly infused with even more life. Eternal life, if you will. Not a life that lasts forever and ever in a fairytale land, but an ordinary, everyday life made transcendent even in the most mundane moments—as if the Creator himself were present in them.

My faith has allowed me the freedom to make every moment count. And when you are ticking off the moments like opening windows on an advent calendar, that is no small thing.

CHAPTER 3
Theatre of ups and downs

On November 15, 2010, I finally became a doctor.

For me, medicine is more than a vocation, it is an intellectual challenge, it is a passion—but above all, it is the chance to serve humanity when they are at their most weak, their most frail, and their most mortal. The privilege to input into people's lives during these moments cannot be understated, and with it comes responsibility, respect and reverence for the human condition.

It should not be forgotten that it is in light of our suffering, our brokenness, and our trials and tribulations that our accomplishments, our joy and our celebrations become all the more colourful. Life is a vivid theatre of ups and downs; each up is only as monumental as the down that precedes it. It is in light of cancer that I can celebrate this achievement with so much more vigour.

'Qualification', The Boredom Blog, November 19, 2010

I understand why people who know they are about to die often question the purpose and value of their lives, even down to questioning who they are, or who they have been. I do not question those things about my own life, but I have experienced how death strips away the layers of identity you have spent a lifetime forming. Even the photo of me up on the wall looks nothing like who I am now. I am barely recognisable, even to myself. And I am told that I do not laugh like I used to, and that my short spells of low mood are out of character. I gave up my position in the hospital months ago. My blog posts have been sporadic for most of this year. It feels as though, at the end, the achievements that have marked your life and set you apart have been set to one side. One thing only remains—the end itself. So who am I at the end? Or perhaps this is a better way of saying it: what is left of the person I have been? The husband of Hannah? The son of Royston and Ruth? Elise's father?

My parents are constant visitors to the house. Mum has been a nurse and does far more for me than any mother should have to do for a son at this stage of his life. No parent expects their child to go before them. They expect to spend their lives celebrating the milestones of their children's lives—things like award nights and graduations. My parents have been there for those things, events that helped to carve out my identity and purpose in this world, if only for a brief time. They are the moments that seem to say as much about the parent as they do the child. Moments of pride, satisfaction and fulfilment. A job well done. Moments to capture in photos and post online so that friends and family can share in the joy.

Parents certainly do not expect to be visiting the home of their son as he counts down the final moments of his life in the sure knowledge that there are, at most, just a couple of weeks to go.

We do not talk about this, though, my parents and I. Though present on the journey and intimately involved in the stark realities of what dying is actually like for me, they are on their own path—and need to be. Theirs is a different journey to mine. Difficult in its own way, for sure. Devastating, no doubt. Theirs is a type of loss I will never have to experience. But it is a path they have to follow and endure together— without me.

I posted a picture of the three of us online—me, Royston and Ruth—after my graduation. It was one of the biggest moments of my life, the fulfilment of a long, long journey, and one I was not sure I would ever complete. Parents stand beside you at graduation ceremonies because they have walked with you through the formative years. They are beside you in your early days of school, in your confused teen years, in the struggles after high school when you think you know what direction you will take, and then when you change your mind and become utterly muddled. The times you have no money, no clue, no drive. All these moments are reflected in their smiles on that night. And in mine, too. A smile that is so big, so proud and so mindful of what I have been able to achieve, with no small amount of grace.

On the day I finished med school, I cried as I walked to the bus stop to head home. I had made it. And I could not believe it. I am not given to dramatic tears, but on this occasion they came in response to an overwhelming sense of disbelief—I had just completed my last year of a medical degree against all the odds. I always knew that finishing med school would be a massive achievement, in and of itself. It is for anyone who completes it. But I had finished my final year while undergoing chemo- therapy. Just one year before, I was told my cancer was terminal. That was the same month I sat and watched as my colleagues, the cohort with whom I had started my degree and with whom I had spent nights in the library working on assignments and studying for exams, graduated from med school before me.

Yet here I was. Finished. Walking for the bus, heading home, about to become a doctor. Surreal, for sure. Emotional, definitely. It was not meant to happen. But it had.

Was the moment bittersweet, knowing as I did that not even graduation would remove the reality of my terminal disease? I do not remember now. What I remember is that there was not really the time to think about my sickness. As soon as I was sure I would live long enough to finish my degree—and by this I literally mean, once I was staring down the barrel of qualification—I approached the hospital to line up a position. Two weeks later, I was on the job. I worked a sixteen-hour shift that first day, a sign of things to come. I did my first lumber puncture and it worked. I came home. I was hot. I was sweaty. The adrenaline was still pumping. And I was energised. I had just finished my first day as a doctor, overwhelmingly happy. I can taste the high of that moment, even now.

It was scary, definitely. And every experience was heightened by the struggles of the previous two years since Diagnosis Day. Every sense was primed by the depths of disappointment I had experienced, then the highs of the achievement. And then there was the job itself. Suddenly, you are writing prescriptions for the first time. You are giving life-altering advice and putting your name to it. And that is the thing. You are putting your name to someone's wellbeing. Giving that person everything you are, so that they can be well—so that they can become everything they can be.

I had discovered who I was. I was Dr Jared Noel.

I have heard people describe the process by which we are formed as 'people' as a relational achievement, meaning that our identity is as much a result of the relationships we are in as it is of any individual qualities or talents. This is very true in my case. And the 'achievement' of becoming a doctor was many years in the making. I am talking about more than study and the process of qualifying with a degree. The journey towards becoming a doctor began in my youth, and it involved the formation of my spiritual calling as much as it did my training and vocational preparation. And there were some missteps along the way.

If, at the age of eight or nine, my idea of what I would be later in life was fairly clichéd, by my teen years I had developed a pretty good idea. If someone had asked me at the age of around fourteen, I would have said three things: archaeologist, forensic scientist or doctor. I was aware at school that I was doing pretty well—notwithstanding those rough years I have alluded to, which had more to do with the family's regular relocation than inability or poor performance. I was never anything other than pretty much top of the class in school, but how much work I put in to be at the top depended on the class and the teacher. These were the beginnings of me being aware of my need for extrinsic motivation. As I progressed through high school I knew that I was not arty—at all! And while I played music I was not actually a musician. I started playing the piano from around the age of ten and then picked up the violin around thirteen. On reflection, I wish my parents had told me not to pick up the violin but to pick up the guitar. It is a much cooler instrument.

I was also aware that I enjoyed science and had an inquisitive mind—I had known this for years, which is why I eventually became two of the three things on my wish list. I have not yet had the opportunity to be an archaeologist. And I am afraid that no amount of being at the top of the class can achieve that now.

But by the time I finished secondary studies, I was not that sure anymore. I had my ideas, but I lacked conviction either way. I applied for med school, but more out of being smart enough to do it, and because I had friends who were doing it. As it happened, my application was rejected, so I decided on a Bachelor of Science because it was the obvious area of study for me to pursue. I came back to the city for university, and my parents decided to come back too—much to my disappointment, as I was looking forward to the student life on my own. But at least living at home was cheaper than flatting.

My trip to the Philippines coincided with the end of my second year in science. And just a few months later I submitted my second application to med school, in the hope that I could begin at the end of my science degree. I had become passionate about the idea of doing medicine overseas. To me, it seemed the most logical way of pursuing the vision that was gaining more clarity all the time. But my application was rejected this time as well.

That left forensic science, a course that is harder to get into than med school these days. And I remember walking away from that interview knowing it was where I was meant to be. I did not know why, and I could not reconcile this with my vision of working overseas—the two things just did not seem to fit—but I just knew. And I got in. In hindsight, forensics is where I found myself, and where I learnt about my capacity to battle through dark days. And this was vital for what was about to happen.

When I finished my undergraduate degree I continued on to a Master of Science, majoring in forensic science. Academically, this was a smooth period of my life. Personally, it was not the case. And I reflect on this now only because what I learnt during this time, and learnt about myself, shaped who I would be as a doctor and how I would handle my own sickness. It also affirmed my belief that it is often through the darkest times that you learn the most—that is, if you acknowledge those struggles for what they are and avoid the temptation to whitewash them with shallow philosophies.

I was between churches at the time, which is significant because it meant my primary group of friends were the people who were doing the degree with me. My closest friend—the one I said goodbye to just a week ago—had been a youth leader at the church I attended through my undergraduate years, and this had been the context in which I had found a community, and that had been so formative in my passion for overseas work. When he left the church, I did, too. The people I chose to hang out with instead were my fellow students—and it turned out they were not the best people to be with. Some friendships you make in life turn out to be more destructive and toxic than is good for you, nice enough people though they might be. I discovered for the first time how damaging this could be for me personally. I also discovered the harsh reality that ending certain relationships is the only way you can move forward.

Significantly, though, it plunged me into severe depression—clinical depression. I was confronted with my own limitations, the tough realities of loneliness and isolation, and the discovery of what being an extrovert meant in terms of my need for people and community, solid friendships that helped to stabilise and normalise me. Without these sorts of relationships I could not function in any kind of meaningful way. It was also a stark reminder of the reality of suffering and my own dependence on spiritual solutions to dark times like these, as well as on the typical pharmaceutical solutions. I took antidepressants for a time, but it was as much my own reflection and soul-searching, not to mention the spiritual disciplines I had been raised with, that helped me through.

In hindsight, this whole season happened because of a series of things that converged to make me just very, very sad about life. Destructive friendships and disappointments with people I held in great esteem turned my life upside down. Essentially, I was discovering that life did not always go the way it was 'meant to'. The outcome for me was that I cut ties with people I found destructive, and I intentionally sought a community I could belong to. And this coincided with the completion of my masters.

At twenty-three, I had finished two degrees and had begun a career in forensic science, specialising in DNA profiling. Some formative months overlap at this stage in my story. I worked full-time as a forensic scientist for a year, then continued part-time for several years when I eventually entered med school. The depression lasted about two years, and while some would not consider that long compared to the years and years others battle depression, it felt much longer at the time. I was in the depths of that dark place for nine months to a year, and did not start to emerge until after a good eighteen months. I continued my studies through this time. And while words such as 'darkness' are apt for such periods, ironically they produce a lot of light—for me, some real insight into how I think, how I ended up at the bottom, what I need to do well in life. It also made me robust, and without it my approach to my current circumstances might have been quite different.

And behind the scenes, of course, something else was happening that would have more of an impact than studies, or depression, or destructive relationships. I already had cancer. I did not know it, of course. I would not discover it for several years yet. But, most likely, those cells were already mutating, already multiplying aggressively in ways that would not produce symptoms for some time.

I cannot help but wonder, what if I had known? The reality is, there was no way of knowing without some sort of investigative procedure. And on the basis of nothing symptomatic, no doctor was ever going to investigate. So, I think back with a sense of the irony of it more than anything.

In the midst of all this came my decision to go to med school. Or, at least, to try for a third time to get in. And this decision came out of the blue. At the time, life was starting to work. All the pieces were in place. I was working full-time. I was a forensic scientist. I was flatting. I was finally free of my university years. I had an income, which was nice. But there was this one thing. I still held strongly to my conviction that I was being called to the Third World. I just could not figure out how on earth forensics was going to get me there. I had been overseas several times since that first trip to the Philippines. I was a firm believer in the idea that if you have been given such a strong vision as the one I was carrying, it is up to you to stoke the fire and keep it alive. If you fail to put wood on it, ten years will have gone by and you will find nothing but ashes and charred embers. So, I had travelled ever since that initial sense of calling took shape, keeping the hunger alive and looking for opportunities to pursue my goal.

But here I was, a fresh graduate, with money for the first time in my life, no longer living in below-par student accommodation and with no more arguments about whose turn it was to do the dishes. But I had no idea how God was going to reconcile this lifestyle, and this career, with that clear calling—a calling that was clear to me, anyway. And by now this calling had become more than a desire to work with underprivileged people. It was already who I was. It was an identity.

I had given up on the dream of med school at this stage. It was no longer in my mind that medicine might be the avenue by which I would get overseas. I had done five years of university already and the idea of going back there for another five years of med school was ludicrous. When the idea came to me, one morning while I was reflecting quietly by myself, it came from nowhere. It is still clear in my mind. It was the middle of winter. I was going through my usual morning routine. I was reading, probably. Perhaps some prayer. But it may as well have been an audible voice, the impression was so strong—just like the time I was baptised. The voice was direct: 'Apply for med school.' My response: 'Really? That dream is over.' So I thought about it some more. And then some more. And, I admit, I found the idea interesting. While it was a dream I had given up on, it was a dream I had been passionate about. In my mind at the time, there was no doubt this was the same God who had told me to own my faith when I was a teenager. In the ten years since that first conviction I had not heard the voice again, but I remembered it so well, I did not even question the wisdom of what I believed I was being told to do. So I looked into the application process and found out the deadline was a week away. My previous attempts had been submitted at the end of each year, but this year the process had been brought forward by six months. Still, I made the deadline—just. And the application resulted in an interview, further than I had ever got before. And the interview led to an admission, and suddenly my life was on the verge of a complete transformation. I was going back to university, back to being a student, but this time I was going to be studying medicine.

I have reflected many times on why I was successful this time and not the others. There were practical reasons, of course. I was a postgrad, which meant I was applying under a different category. It also meant that I began my medical studies as a second-year student. I had obtained my masters degree with first-class honours, which significantly bumped up my grade-point average. But this time there was a spiritual difference. I was convinced of it. I know that colleagues who do not share my faith would be sceptical about this component, but for me it was the key difference between this application and the other two. The first time I applied because I could; the second time because I wanted to; the third time because I was told to. This time it was not so much a feeling that I was doing something for God but that I was obeying. My sense of this at the time, and even now, was profound. And, of course, in the back of my mind was the vision and how this now made sense. To me, it was the resolution of the calling, and the resurrection of the dream.

I say that I am not given to tears, but here at the very beginning of a journey that would culminate in my eventual qualification as a doctor, I also found myself in tears. I remember that day I received the letter telling me I had an interview with med school. Just an interview! I was home from work for lunch, fortunately. I opened the letter and was immediately hit by its significance. This was an invitation to re-dream the dream.

And I cried.

———————

Med school was quite a different experience to anything I had known before. Collegially, academically, competitively, this was a different league. It made even my previous masters studies feel like a walk in the park. I went straight into second year in 2005, joining a cohort of around 160 students. Ahead of me were two years of pre-clinical studies—theory-based lectures, mainly—followed by three years of clinical programs—hospital-based studies that ready you for practice as a doctor. I remember the first two years as intense times. The bar was raised so high, just to pass a course. The standard required to beat your fellow students was even higher. Competitiveness is one of my core traits. It manifested at med school as me having to know how well everyone else was doing so I knew how well I was doing in comparison, and how well I needed to do to be above average. And that is not easy when everyone is operating at such a high level. You are all sitting the same papers for a start, so it is like you are running the same race. This is great for building cama-raderie and serious friendships that last a lifetime. There was a sense from the beginning that we were all in this together. For someone like me, who had discovered in the recent past how brutal a lack of collegiality could be, this was a key aspect of this period. The workload was intense from my very first year. But when you are still in the library at eight o'clock on a Friday night, and all your friends are there too, there is something very cool about the demands of the course. There is a massive sense of achievement, for one thing. And in this a solidarity is formed, which you carry into the workplace when you all grad-uate together.

As you begin your clinical years, the sense begins to build of how good you can be as a doctor, and that this is no arbitrary thing but the actual difference between life and death for some people. I went from wanting to be the best possible student, to wanting to be the best possible doctor. And not for the sake of competition, but for the sake of people who were sick and suffering. Behind this was always that sense of greater purpose, that, for me, med school was now the route God would use to take me into the developing world. There was a context for the calling now, and the further I went in my studies, the more sharply defined that vision became. It did not matter to me that I was studying again, and yet again without money. The promise of a greater salary at the end of my studies was not a factor either. My eye was on the goal, and day by day, course by course, the goal was getting closer.

I had completed two years of clinical studies before my cancer diagnosis, at the end of the fifth year of my medical degree. Those two years had given me plenty of opportunity to consider what fields of medicine I would move into in order to practise overseas. I travelled during this time too, just to gain experience of life and culture, even medical practices, in the developing world. I spent time in general medicine, general practice, surgery—your studies expose you to the many possible specialties you can practise within those fields. Those years honed in me my sense of calling, as I put into practice what I had done all this learning for. Some days I would come home exhausted, realising the work I had done all day was neither fun nor invigorating. And that is how I would work out that a particular field of medicine was not for me. Other days I would come home just as exhausted but also energised. The surgical specialties did this for me, and while I remained open to any number of possibilities, not wanting to foreclose on anything, I knew I could happily spend a lifetime as a general surgeon. And I knew that in the places where I wanted to make a difference, surgeons were often hard to find and particularly valuable.

There was another upshot to those first two clinical years. By the time I was diagnosed with cancer I had intimate knowledge of the very hospital where that diagnosis was made. I knew the processes and systems, how things worked. I had seen people diagnosed with similar things, and worse things, and witnessed how foreign the experience could be for them. For me, it was not a foreign experience at all.

It is fair to say I loved med school. I loved my clinical training. And I loved work. If it is true that you are what you love, then medicine was my niche. At the core of this love was the doctor–patient interaction, and the opportunities you are given daily to make a difference in someone's life. As you progress through your career you get more and more of these opportunities. Even as a student, there are moments when you get to do things you know are significant—in among all the times you spend observing another doctor's work practices and feel somewhat superfluous. The satisfaction for me was not in watching someone else, but in actually playing a role. Actually changing a person's life. And that is what medicine is about. And that was my calling. As a doctor, you are in a privileged position, invited into someone's life—often at times that are emotionally dark for them—and given the opportunity to make all the difference.

One patient comes to mind now, as she has over the years. I am not sure why I have thought about her so often, because I do not even know whether I made a difference. I was not even involved in her treatment. She was just someone I observed in emergency once, and whose situation touched something in me. It was after my diagnosis, I remember that—so perhaps something of her vulnerability has stayed with me.

She was a meth addict, around 21 years old, suffering withdrawal. The emergency department is not the place to go to for acute withdrawal, so they could not really treat her. Her addiction was so bad that she had been injecting meth into the spaces beneath her fingernails, because she had destroyed all her veins everywhere else. She had been through rehab more than once, without any success. So here she was, in emergency, wracked by the symptoms of acute withdrawal. She was a victim of her own decisions as much as anything, for sure, yet no longer really the product of those decisions, but rather of the drug addiction itself. She was curled up on the bed in the foetal position, sweating and convulsing. As the doctor was dealing with her, a compulsion came over me to take a step back and pray. That rarely happens for me. Even as a person of faith, when it comes to medicine I am very pragmatic. And so this occasion has always stood out. Why I felt that then, I do not know. And I have no idea what happened to her or whether she is even alive. I just know that my heart was suddenly filled with compassion for her.

With love, even. Or a form of it.

———————

The vision that took on even greater definition on that mid-winter morning many years ago gave immense purpose and drive to the years that followed. I thought at the time that was all about medicine and working on behalf of suffering, sick and underprivileged people in the developing world. As it turned out, it was as much about my need as theirs. I still have questions about why the call was so clear when things were not going to go that way. I brought those questions home with me when I came back from the hospice four weeks ago. They have stuck with me during these weeks of steady and gradual deterioration, and now as I fight the fatigue to finish these reflections. They are not questions that plague or frustrate me, but they are unresolved.

Some people would argue that subjective impressions of a spiritual nature are always flawed. Perhaps I heard the call wrongly. Perhaps there was no call at all. Perhaps there is no God. How can a man of science pin his hopes and his dreams and build a life around some mystical call to action?

Most of my colleagues would be atheists—this often happens as a result of the med-school system itself—it is hard to maintain a faith in the face of science—but even so, I think most people can relate to some sort of faith component in their lives. As a scientist, yes, it is almost a mutually exclusive thing to say that I am a physician on the one hand, but to hold faith so tightly in the other. Faith, which is not evidence-based at all, and which can appear quite airy-fairy, seems to be a crutch for vulnerable and susceptible people. And putting faith in an entity that can never be tested . . . it is a big leap to take when you have based your identity and purpose on knowable quantities.

But in my experience, working with both doctors and patients, you would be hard-pressed to find anyone who would not allow for some form of faith component in their lives. Sometimes they acknowledge it exists but do not know how to describe it. Or they cannot fathom how it works out in their own lives because it is this other thing that is not fostered or nurtured. So, it is just a thing they have, but one they do not understand. Most people have this thing. If it is not couched in the language of faith or religion, it is often couched in new-age philosophies or pseudoscientific beliefs about the universe, or contemplative practices and meditative techniques, or even psychological tools such as visualisation. For some, such as me, it is couched in the language of Christian faith, or variations of the faith. But at some level there is a component of faith in how most people engage in knowledge and the questions we have— about life itself, or about relationships, or meaning, or love. For me, my understanding of that day comes from the faith tradition I have already described. And in that framework I heard it as a direction, a call to serve—and a call to prepare myself for service by going to med school, in spite of my past failures at admission. I also heard it as a call to achieve great things, not just by working as a surgeon but by challenging the status quo, to shake the powers and authorities who were keeping people shackled in situations of poverty.

As I progressed through med school, and even later when I went into the practice of medicine itself, I was honing this vision, working to understand myself in the context of medicine so that I could move into that overseas setting. I spent two months in India during this time, then three months in the Philippines. I needed to find out whether I was able to spend such lengthy stints in those places, to demonstrate to myself that I could. In the Philippines I did mainly pastoral and relief-response work, distributing clothing up into the mountains. I took kilos of clothing from New Zealand. A year later, I spent two months in India, and one of those I spent in a hospital. Again, I wanted to experience the actual practice of medicine in a context similar to one in which I might ultimately end up. As it happened, this month was not particularly helpful, for the simple reason that my training was not yet advanced enough to make the most of it. But still, my heart was always leaning in this direction. As to where this work might go, I was still open. My experience had been in South-East Asia, so I was always being drawn back there, but Africa was in the back of my mind.

By the time I was a postgrad, working in the hospital full time, my desire to become a general surgeon had been cemented. Of course, by this stage the cancer had advanced. I knew that I was terminal, and that in all likelihood I had two years to live, but I managed to work from the end of 2010 to the end of 2013—three years. By the time it became obvious that I could no longer carry on working to the required standard, I had been offered a pathway through the hospital that would have realised my dream. Relinquishing this dream was one of the hardest things I have ever done in my life.

Before I ended my career as a doctor, I was awarded the Confederation of Postgraduate Medical Education Councils Junior Doctor of the Year Award. There is a recipient from each state in Australia and one from New Zealand. I did not deserve the award, if I am honest. It is given for engagement with other doctors, involvement in ongoing learning, and commitment to the values of what it is to be a doctor. I guess it is based on what they think truly represents the idea of being a doctor. It was a humbling experience to receive this, but I do not know any doctor who would take it and say they deserved it. As far as I am concerned, I have worked with doctors around me who do a better job, or at least are better at their job than I am. Nevertheless, I include the award with all those other things occurring in my life that added to my growing appreciation that I was at least fulfilling a bigger mission. The award, as well as comments from colleagues and the reactions from patients, helped me realise that I was actually living out this vision, and that I was pretty good at it, too. In that respect, receiving the award was an honour.

But fuelling my passion more than anything was my belief that I was following a specific direction and fulfilling my life's calling. And that was why it was so hard to give it up. I felt that I was giving up the very thing God had asked me to do. Giving up on God, in a way. By giving me that calling, God had given me an identity—that of a doctor. The reality is, no one goes into medicine thinking it is just a job. When your title changes, it marks the identity shift that goes along with it, and how much you are now required to immerse yourself in the role.

So, as I think back to my tears at finishing the degree, it was about far more than the satisfaction of completing my studies. This, as far as the milestones of my life go, was fundamental in shaping who I was. Shaping Jared. And when my work was eventually taken away, in late 2013, just three years later, a large part of my self was already wrapped up in what I had become. Dr Noel. When it went, my identity seemed to go with it.

And yet . . . there was a new sense of self just around the corner, one that was very much linked to Elise and her arrival in the world.

All I had to do was survive long enough to experience it.

CHAPTER 4
All the clichés

Hannah has been all the clichés you can think of: the wind beneath my wings, the person who makes me better, the person who completes me . . . the list goes on. Clichés only faintly touch on what words cannot even express about what she means to me, and how supportive she has been to me over the last fourteen months of life.

So today I want to honour Hannah. I want to acknowledge the fact that cancer is not a diagnosis that only affects the individual with the disease, it affects the family unit as well. People often comment to me about how I have dealt with this adversary, but truth be told, Hannah's strength is 80 per cent of the source of my courage. She is the one to be honoured today. She is the one who needs to be remembered in your prayers as much as me. I might be the one with cancer, but it is us together who battle it.

'To Hannah', The Boredom Blog, January 12, 2010

I have slept in two beds during these last weeks at home. I say slept, but what I mean is that I spend the day here. Day and night. Apart from those brief times I have spent downstairs. Right now I am in the bed I share with Hannah, propped up on pillows. There is a plastic carton beside my leg in case I vomit, and a bag of lollies beside that to take away the awful taste in my mouth—and to give me a sugar boost when I need one. There is a magazine, propped open at a favourite page. My iPhone is here, too. It receives a steady stream of text messages throughout the day, mainly from friends wondering how I am in the moment. I suspect they can tell by my silence that I am not at my best. I have responded less and less to these good wishes as the days have ticked away. They will all be answered at some stage—but by Hannah, not by me. The main use I have for the phone now is to text Hannah, who is downstairs, to let her know when I need more pain relief. Being married to a medical doctor is an advantage when it comes to dying at home.

The other bed in the room is the one where I have spent most of my time. It is a hospital bed, borrowed from the local hospice, and the family were able to fit it between this bed and the corner of the room to my right. It is raised higher than this one. There is enough space between the two to fit a small metal table, on which the family has placed a jug of water and a glass. In my first days back in the house I spent more of my time there. During the day, the windows behind my head were opened to let the breeze blow through. Despite the end being so close, the freshness of the room reflected a freshness in the way I felt about confronting this last challenge, from this place. Our home. Our room. I will probably die in that bed. When the time comes.

It was a shock when, on my second evening home, I fell out of that bed and crashed onto the small metal table. I had lost so much of my strength during the weeks I was in the hospital that I was unable to get back up. This was a new thing for me. The family came in, of course, and everything was okay. There were no injuries, other than to my pride. But the reality of my situation hit me quite forcefully—I had deteriorated to such an extent that I could not even hold my balance in the way I once could. I was merely reaching to take something from the table, but did not factor in the loss of my core strength and the weakness of my thighs and hips. With no strength in my lower half to maintain balance, over I went. It was a moment of realisation. Another one. I realised there was no coming back from this. I was going downhill, quickly. And this was a hill I would not be climbing back up. I set a new target for myself after that. I would rehab my legs, work at regaining some of the strength I had lost so I could at least move about the house. And I did achieve that. But never did I think my situation was going to improve again.

That night comes to mind now, as I think of Hannah and how different these past years would have been without her. How differently I would have confronted my illness and what challenges I would have faced were she not here beside me. In truth, there are challenges that I have faced because she *is* here and *is* sharing this journey with me. These are challenges I would have missed out on but that have taught me things about myself I never would have confronted were she not part of the picture. Like how to live in the presence of love in the way I have been forced to. Like how to live in a place of vulnerability that I never once envisaged as being part of my life. The truth is, I was embarrassed when I fell out of bed. I was ashamed that I had lost even the ability to hold myself upright. That I had become the patient. That Hannah and her mother had to lift me up from the floor and back into bed. And that Hannah was seeing me deteriorate. This was not on offer when I asked Hannah to marry me. It was never what I intended for her.

But I have come to know more about Hannah in the context of sickness, and now in the process of dying. The different phases of our relationship have been about discovery in their own ways. Courtship, early marriage, then marriage post-diagnosis, family life—and now dying. And while this vulnerability is the toughest thing I have faced, the past six years have been about discovering the great capacity of love to reach into any situation of suffering and generate hope. And in that I have discovered that while Hannah is 'all the clichés', I could not have shared this adventure with anyone more capable, more understanding or more trusting.

Even so, my death will rob us of a vision we have shared since the very first time we met, huddled around a fire waiting for breakfast, two young Kiwis out there in the world, champing at the bit to make a difference.

———————

I knew Hannah was special from our first conversation. She must have been, because it was a conversation I did not want to end. So it lasted an entire day, then the next day, too. And somewhere along the way, I knew she was a woman I could spend my life with. But subsequent years have made me appreciate just how perfect she was for me and for what we would experience together. My feelings about this, though, are now complicated by the regrets I have about inviting her into this particular marriage. We had barely a year of 'normality' before my diagnosis, and I will leave her soon to pursue dreams that we have only talked about. At the same time, she has been the reason I have achieved so much in these past few years. She was there when I graduated, when I finished my first day of work, each time I received bad news from an oncologist, each and every time I was brought to tears by the loss of more hope. She was the right person for me before I got sick. From the perspective that came later, I knew that even more. Committed. Strong. Loyal. Passionate. Patient. Words we over-use and mis-use to communicate small things tend not to be adequate when you want to express something as big as what I want to say about Hannah. But they are the right words. And read in the context of what happened to us, they recover their significance. A year after becoming my wife on the back of dreams we shared at our first meeting, Hannah is suddenly the wife of a cancer patient. A year later, she knows the cancer is terminal. If she is lucky, she might get to have two more years with me, and those two years dominated by chemotherapy. Certainly not what we imagined.

But she has stood by my side. More than that, she has been on this journey the whole time. She has taken every step, in sync with my own. She has lent me her strength. She has helped me cope. She has supported my work, rejoiced in the new opportunities that have presented themselves in the face of my illness, and wept with me each time there has been more bad news to hear. She is the key to how I have managed so well, the subtext to the blogs I have posted online.

And in recent months I have discovered something more in her: the qualities she has as a mother—despite her fears about how good she would be. Disciplined, caring, imaginative, doting. Again, adjectives are not adequate. Let me say it like this: I have no fear about how great she will be as a mum in my absence.

We met one morning in 2006 in the Blue Mountains, outside Sydney, Australia, while most other conference delegates slept in line with their own time zones. Used to rising a couple of hours before Australians living on the east coast, we Kiwis were up first, and I met Hannah sitting beside the fire before breakfast was even served. It was the International Christian Medical and Dental Association World Congress, an event that happens every four years, so I knew before we started talking that Hannah was probably a Christian and also working in medicine. It did not take us long to establish that we not only had those things in common, we also shared some key values, the same nationality, similar church backgrounds, and a vision for where we hoped to take our work. I had been on my second trip to the Philippines just six months before, and she had already done a medical elective in Nepal. She was open to travel and adventure, and shared my ideas about mission work, the underprivileged and working in contexts completely different from the privileged world in which we had been raised. So, as we sat there in the freezing cold, in the middle of winter, June 2006, we shared with each other our dreams.

Hannah was ahead of me in medicine, despite me being a year older. She was already working, having gone straight to med school from secondary school. I was in my second year of med school (the third year of the degree). She was already earning, while I was still raising sponsorship to enable me to do my overseas trips. After chatting by the fire for a couple of hours, we had breakfast together. Then throughout that day the conversation progressed as we attended the same sessions and caught up in the times between. The next day was the same. The details are hazy now, but I am blaming the Fentanyl— my pain relief—rather than the typical faulty memory for romantic moments that husbands often have. I do remember that it all developed quite quickly. By the end of the day we had built up a good understanding of each other—our stories and backgrounds, the things we were passionate about, the values instilled in us in the ways we were brought up. And when the conference was over, we exchanged contact details. She was heading back to Dunedin in the South Island, I was heading back to Auckland in the North. But I do remember that the very next day, I sent her an email that said if she was ever in Auckland to let me know and I would take her out for dinner. She answered by saying she had some leave soon and would fly up. It was the easiest date I ever got.

So our relationship began, from either end of the country. It was six weeks before Hannah would come to Auckland, and in that time our relationship developed by email and texts and telephone calls. Our first actual date in person was six weeks down the track, well after the relationship had begun. It was clear to me even then that Hannah was unlike anyone I had met before. And to me, it was clear that I could see myself sharing my life with her. This was significant for me—I had worked out pretty early on in other relationships that I could not spend a lifetime with them. But it was strange to me, as well. I never imagined I would be with an introvert such as Hannah. And what set her apart from other girls I had known was an intangible quality, something I could not name at the time, and perhaps still can't. There was just something different. A depth, perhaps. Maybe it was the God factor. Much of it had to do with personality, and the complementary sense of our differences but how we agreed on key dreams and goals. I had not anticipated these things in the person I pictured would be my wife. But how we wanted to live our lives, what we hoped to achieve, the values that we had set, and the goals we wanted to reach—we came together around those fundamental things.

By the end of that year it was clear to both of us that the relationship was serious. My ongoing vision of working overseas would take me to India for two months over the summer break, and Hannah had made changes, too. She was working in the capital, Wellington, but if our relationship was going to progress towards marriage we at least needed to see whether we could live in the same city first. I was stuck in Auckland completing my studies, so Hannah decided to move close to me. I returned from India as she moved up from Wellington, and our first bona fide year of courtship began. It was all leading to an engagement, obviously. And midway through that year, the first anniversary of our meeting in Australia, I proposed.

I have already alluded to the fact that I am competitive. So there is little point denying that while I had heard some great engagement stories, I was determined to beat them. People have accused me, in subsequent years, of doing this mainly for my own amusement. Which is not entirely true. I wanted Hannah to have a great engagement story to tell. I have also alluded to my pragmatism, and this was evident as the date approached of the anniversary of our meeting in Australia. We'd had conversations about the future, clearly, and I wanted to arrange a dinner on our anniversary but without raising Hannah's expectations, so I told her not to have any. We would go out to dinner to mark our anniversary, but I warned her not to think anything was going to happen—that way, if nothing did happen, she would not be disappointed, and would not forever remember the dinner in a negative light. To be honest, she was a bit gutted about this. But she did come to me the next day and thank me—she would have gone to the dinner with expectations, she admitted, but I had ensured that she could enjoy the dinner without any feelings of being let down. I knew that the proposal itself would make up for any hurt she might feel in the meantime.

The engagement took place over an entire day, and involved much collusion, many balloons, no small amount of planning (weeks, actually), flights, a resort, a beauty spa and dinner. And separate rooms. Which was expensive—but we had conservative Christian values, after all. The first part of the day happened while Hannah was out with a friend, which I had prearranged. I was in her flat, filling it with balloons and with an envelope containing a mystery diagnosis she would have to solve on her return. She would need to consult a medical dictionary I had borrowed at the last minute from the university library, the relevant pages of which concealed an envelope of instructions that directed her to pack and make her way to the airport. I have no idea whether or not by this stage her expectations had been raised, but either way, while she was doing this, I was driving out of the city to Rotorua, my childhood home (one of them), to set up for the evening.

My instructions to Hannah were to pack her bags for an evening away, and to include a swimsuit—instructions that she followed, of course. The same friend who had kept her occupied throughout the morning now drove her to the airport, where she was given further instructions and a ticket for a flight down to Rotorua. There was also cash for a taxi at the other end and instructions to head to the Novotel.

It was not until she was in her room that we saw each other for the first time that day. By that stage she had seen the dozen roses that were on her bed. That almost did not happen—it turns out roses are a rare commodity in Rotorua in June—but the hotel managed to find some and had them on the bed for her arrival, with yet another envelope telling her to get ready for a five o'clock pickup. And that was when I knocked on the door and accompanied Hannah to the Polynesian spa, where I swam for an hour while she had a massage.

The proposal itself happened at dinner. I struggle to remember what I said now. The standard words, probably—something along the lines of the effect she had had on my life, the fact I had not met anyone like her. I do remember where it took place, though—an exclusive dining room in the top resort in Rotorua, just her and me alone, with a grand piano in the corner, champagne by the fire, a five-course meal. I got down on one knee between pre-dinner canapés and entrees, and that is when I proposed—early in the evening so that we could relax and enjoy dinner. Which we did, followed by a limousine ride back to the hotel that included a tour through Rotorua—which is a bit of a waste of time when the limo has tinted windows and it is pitch black outside.

Was it all a bit over the top? Not really. Hannah is worth it. It was a memorable day, and she has enjoyed telling the story. And I did not mind raising the bar for my single male colleagues who were yet to take the plunge and would now have to follow in my shadow.

After all, you only get engaged once.

Unless, of course, your husband dies early. But neither of us knew this at the time.

———————

Just six months later, a whole new phase of our life began. We were married in Hannah's home city of Dunedin, a far more traditional place than Auckland. It is rare to find a guy at a Dunedin wedding without a shirt and tie. We were married three days after Christmas, which proved a terrible time of year to ask your poor medical student mates to travel. But it was a nice wedding. A very classical wedding. And without the extravagance of the proposal.

From that moment, married life is divided into pre-diagnosis and post-diagnosis. Pre-diagnosis, those early, settling-in days, lasted just a year. I was in my fourth year of medicine.

We moved into the flat that eventually became the hub of the faith community we became part of, and stayed in the area when it became time to move on. We began marriage as we intended to continue it—with medical careers, a community of friends, church life, and as many outdoor adventures as we could manage. We went on tramps and travelled when we could, something we had always done before we met and were committed to doing together. There was not a lot of time to establish the norms of married life that other couples without sickness might enjoy. That first year of marriage, for anyone, is about a new type of discovery, a period of enjoyment, for sure, but also setting down good patterns—hopefully—and working out where you will settle and which communities you will commit to. We moved from a church community I had been part of for some time to the faith community that gathered in our home. It was a significant move, but not, in our minds, a permanent one.

So, essentially, that first year was a year of planning. Planning for the future, and for taking the steps towards the goals we had formulated from that first breakfast conversation.

Travel, and ultimately adventure, was always going to be part of the picture for us. It was not just that it formed part of those first conversations over shared dreams, it was an important component of our adult lives as individuals. I do not think you grow up in a small town your whole life, get married, and suddenly proclaim, 'Oh, I think God wants us to go to Africa!' We came into marriage with that hope and expectation. We also agreed that to pursue that sort of work in the future meant fuelling the passion, the same approach I had taken for years. We spent some time working in the Australian outback that year, becoming acquainted with the cultural and social challenges that exist in that part of the world. Taking weekends away during that first twelve months was about spending time together but also about nurturing the adventurous spirit that would build towards our future vision. Take a look at any of the photos of us from that time and you will see me in shorts—ever ready for a tramp or a trip. We rarely had a free weekend of doing nothing. And so we formulated our plans for the year's end, and the following year, my trainee intern year. We decided to head away from the city, back to Rotorua, the scene of our engagement. I liked the hospital there, and moving away from the city to do medicine in a town like Rotorua was consistent with our goals. We aimed to work in several cities over the next few years before heading overseas. But before that, before settling into work, we would travel: to Nepal and Tibet, through South-East Asia, the Middle East, climb Kilimanjaro and head into Zambia, where I would take up a brief internship—my first time in Africa.

But our plans were thwarted. Without warning, or at least without the types of symptoms that might indicate something as serious as bowel cancer, life changed. And so began the second period of our marriage. Post-diagnosis. There was no overseas trip, no moving away to Rotorua. For the next year, there was chemotherapy and a suspension of my studies. Later on in the year, at the cessation of my first rounds of chemo, and on the back of the travel insurance we were able to claim against the cancellation of our trip, we headed to South-East Asia. But this was a consolation prize, great as it was. I could suspend only for short bursts the knowledge that I was sick. We went there in the hope that the chemo had successfully treated my cancer and that we would return to good news. But we returned to terrible news—what we call the first relapse.

So we entered a new phase of married life—terminal sickness and the knowledge that all those plans we had made, the goals we had set, and the vision that brought us together, were probably over. I have been asked how a recently married young couple gets through times like these—what do we talk about, how do we process the sadness and loss?—and I never know what to tell them. You just pick yourself up. Or, rather, you pick each other up. You can wallow in it, or you can choose not to. And that is what we chose. Not to wallow. Having a cause or reason to live that drives you certainly helps to relativise something like cancer. And after my terminal diagnosis we decided that I would try to finish my studies. Year three of marriage saw me back at med school while Hannah worked in paediatrics. This brought its own hardships—it is tough to get through exams when chemotherapy has affected your cognition. I could feel the impact of the drugs on my thinking and had to work harder because of it. And yet, we pushed on.

By putting our heads down and our bums up, we got through. And I realised then what a difference it made having a wife who was also medically trained and could understand not only the workload but also the nature of medicine, and the satisfaction you get from the long hours on the job. Had med school been a write-off, and had I not had Hannah to walk alongside me while I finished, life would have taken a very different trajectory.

We have not had a typical marriage. Cancer has made certain of that. But our marriage was never going to be typical. We did not come together over typical hopes and dreams, and had cancer not even entered the story, our journey together would have followed a very atypical route. But there have been typical moments. Or perhaps I should say, there have been windows of normality in which we have been able to make fairly typical decisions. We bought this house in one such window, for reasons as typical as giving a child the type of security a child requires, and also to provide some financial security for Hannah once I am gone. I guess you could say it was an acknowledgement that

I would die in this house. I certainly knew that I would not get to see this particular piece of the dream bear fruit, but I wanted to do whatever I could to care for Hannah beyond this present time.

The prayer I pray most often is this: 'God, when I am not here, you have to look after Hannah. Because I cannot.'

———————

A long battle with cancer changes the nature of a relationship. There is no doubt about that. On chemo, I was barely an active participant in the marriage. I spent five days on the couch and for all of that time Hannah would look after me. This did tend to heighten my appreciation of the times when I was well, and I began to enjoy marriage in those times slightly differently. My first Christmas with Hannah after the terminal diagnosis was in Dunedin with Hannah's parents. Like most things, Christmas was set within a different paradigm for me now. I could not take for granted that I was going to be here for another one. I remember thinking about how forcefully the materialistic world tells you what you should want for Christmas. But in actual fact, what I wanted for Christmas was something no one could offer.

What I wanted was life, of course, and more of it. I wanted normality, to some degree, but I also wanted to be extraordinary. I wanted to achieve great things, and I wanted to achieve those things with Hannah. Most of all, I wanted a marriage that could follow the path towards which we had taken our first tentative steps. I had been diagnosed in the honeymoon period, that newlywed phase when you expect to be protected from the cruel realities of the world so that you can explore love. As a husband I wanted to protect my wife and build her a future.

And I wanted to journey with her—literally. I wanted her to be a part of what I had envisaged for so long. But here again I had to choose the last door first—and just submit to what was. What else could I do? I could not fix anything, despite my instinctive response. Hannah was now stuck on this journey with me. And as it dawned on us how big this thing was actually going to be, the reality of that journey was impossible to deny. It was one of pain and suffering and loss of future—and loss of dreams. At least, it was the loss of my dreams.

This was always the most difficult aspect for me, knowing that I never married Hannah to put her through this. It was always, and has always been, the hardest thing to reconcile.

I have wondered over these last few weeks in the house whether there is anything regarding my marriage left for me to let go of—some reconciliation or resolution, more that I could accept, more of a submission process I could put myself through—but I think it is just the way it is. I know that I did nothing wrong. What I feel is just abiding sorrow, a deep sadness about the things we will not experience. But that is the pain of love. And that is the risk you take when you kneel before a fire with champagne and commit the rest of your life—however long, however short—to this woman who is better for you than anyone you have met before.

When I fell from the bed I felt as vulnerable and needy as I have ever felt. The first through the door was Hannah, who has seen me at my lowest for years now. We are most vulnerable with the people we love the most, because it is with them that we open up our hearts and allow them to see what no one else sees—the fears, the doubts, even the things we feel the most shame about. And it is because of this that we trust them.

———————————

Hannah.

Here are some random things that I have learnt about Hannah—that I am still learning about Hannah—things that come to me as I think about my wife, about what I will miss. Despite us both being doctors, we worked together just the one time. I say together, but I was a medical student and she was the doctor. We, a bunch of students from med school, accompanied her for the day. She and I were already married, which everyone found quite amusing. It was pure chance. And quite funny.

As a doctor, Hannah is diligent. Meticulous. Detailed. She strikes up a great rapport with patients. As a mother, Hannah is comprehensive. Loving. Nurturing. She is more emotional than I am as a parent. Ever the pragmatist, if we have created a routine for sleep times, I am the one who sticks to it. Hannah finds a crying baby difficult to ignore, which is probably a good thing, considering she is training to be a paediatrician.

Hannah likes to get a job done when it needs to be done. I am not so hasty about it. I like to cook, but cleaning . . . not so much. I will put it off, whereas Hannah will get right in and get it done immediately. And that is when I will feel guilty.

We never stop learning in marriage. I am still learning about Hannah. The extent of her perseverance, for example. Her ability to just get the work done. This experience of my illness would break some people, but not Hannah. I do worry about her capacity to hold it all together, but I know she will not break.

I have learnt that marriage is like a big mirror that is held up to you so you can see your failings. In the reflective engagement you have with your partner, you get to see all your characteristics, both good and bad, the qualities and the frailties. Seven years alongside Hannah have helped me discover the things about my character I would probably work on if I had the time.

Hannah has learnt things, too. For this whole period I have watched her work on patience. It has been difficult for her for a million different reasons, but she has been forced to be patient in so many ways—patient with me, with my sickness, with the suspension of some of her own dreams.

Has it been a typical marriage? The circumstances of it have not been typical, but it has been everything a marriage is intended to be. It has been a relationship full of love and grace and forgiveness, and the giving of ourselves to the other. If that is a normal marriage, then that is what we have had.

This evening, we will follow the routine we have established for these final days of our marriage to protect the space that is ours. In many ways, the daylight hours have become all about 'getting the job done', but after seven o'clock, that is our time. Time alone, to talk or to pray or to watch television. Our quality time together. Soon our quality time will be over. The more exhausted I become, the less the word 'quality' seems apt to describe the times we have. And even these times will pass. It will be Hannah alone. Alone with Elise. Hannah will return to work and they will both continue with their lives. These past few years will recede into memory as the years roll on. And Hannah will move on, too. New relationships, new decisions, new goals and dreams.

Was it worth it, in the end? Will Hannah think it was all worthwhile, despite how things have gone? Without a second thought. It was because of our marriage that Elise came to be here. Elise, who has given us so much life. I think of the joy she has given us already, and I know that in those moments when Hannah feels sad and misses the conversation that began over breakfast all those years ago and never actually ended, she only

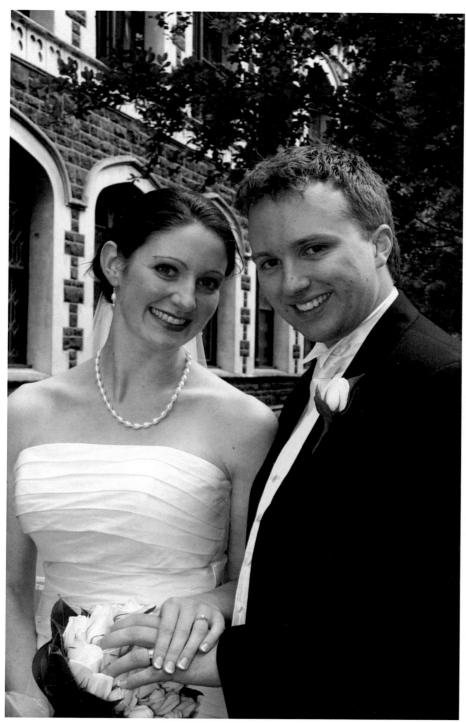

Jared and Hannah on their wedding day, December 28, 2007. KERRY CROSLAND
(KELK PHOTOGRAPHY)

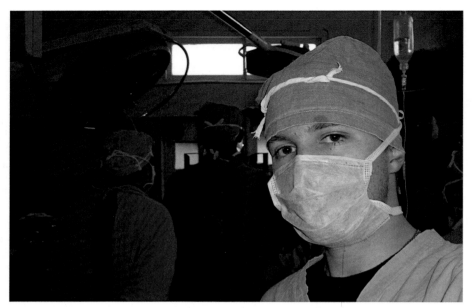

Jared gets some theatre experience in a hospital in India, January 2007.

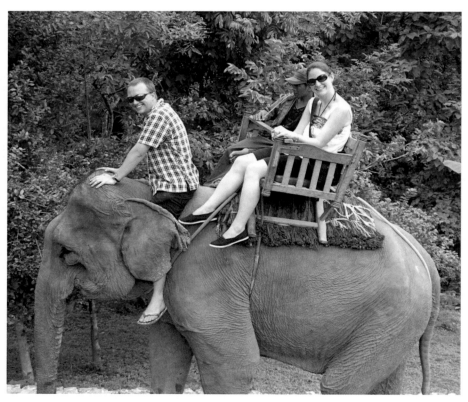

Jared and Hannah elephant riding in Luang Prabang in Laos, October 2009.

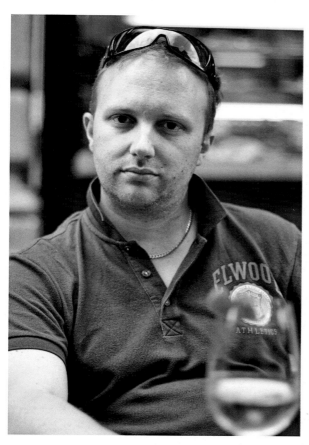

left Jared enjoys lunch at a cafe in Milan, Italy, on September 30, 2012.

below Jared playing with a python on Paradise Island in the Philippines, on September 29, 2009.

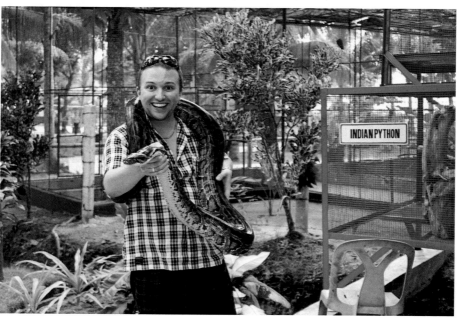

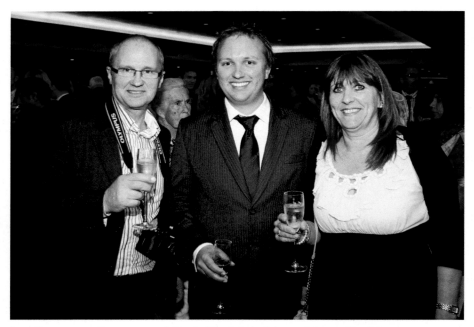

Jared's parents, Royston and Ruth Noel, join him at his medical degree qualification ceremony on November 15, 2010.

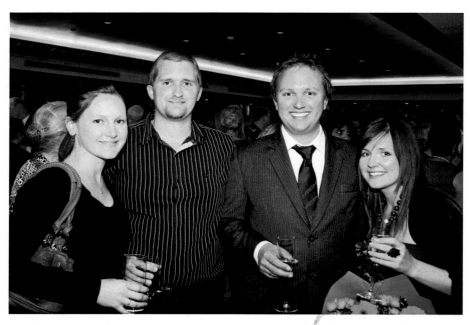

Jared's siblings celebrate his qualification from med school. From left: Sarah and Matt Noel (Jared's brother) and Cara Cameron (Jared's sister).

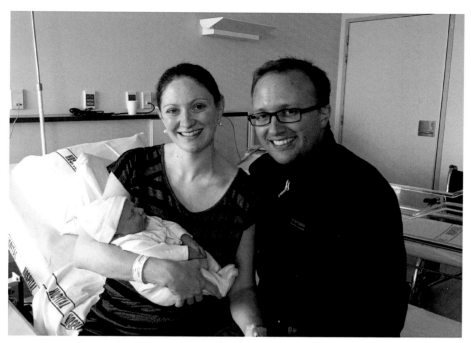

Hannah and Jared welcome Elise Alexandra Grace Noel into the world on January 17, 2014.

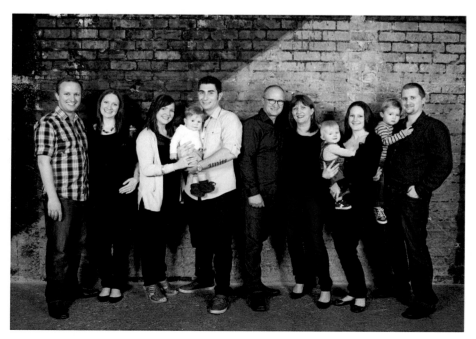

The Noel family prior to Elise's birth, October 2013. KIRSTY HARKNESS (TIGER TIGER PHOTOGRAPHY)

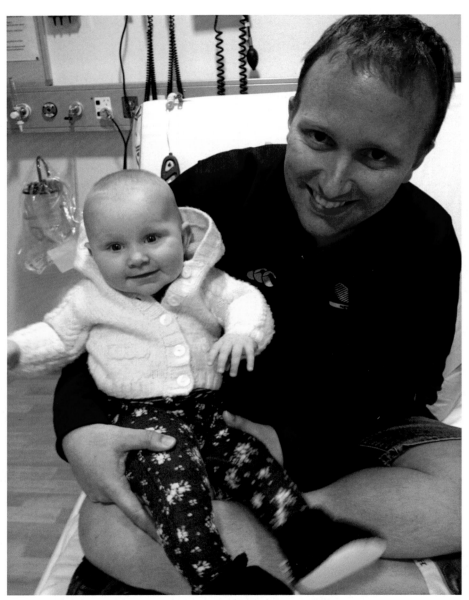

Elise with Jared during his admission to hospital in June 2014.

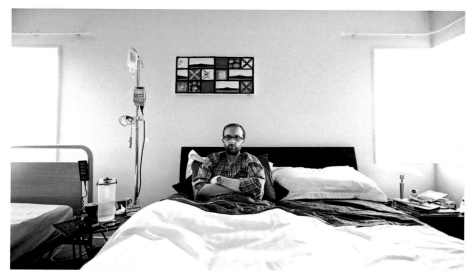

Jared in the room where the conversations for this book took place, September 15, 2014. DAVID W. WILLIAMS

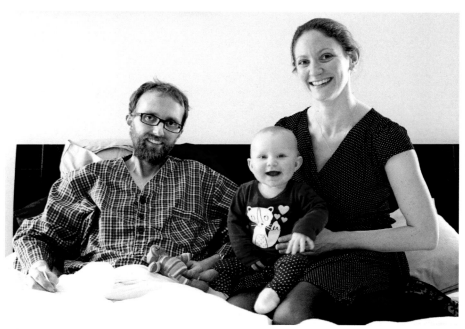

The final family photo taken of Jared, Hannah and Elise, September 24, 2014. DAVID W. WILLIAMS

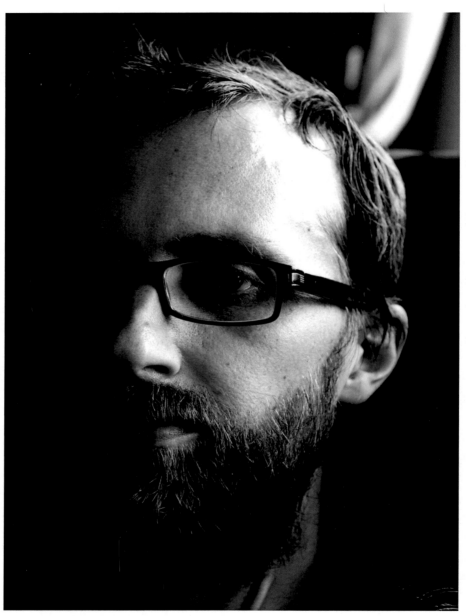

A portrait of Jared taken on a rare day out of bed, relaxing on a recliner rocker in the family room of his home, September 16, 2014. DAVID W. WILLIAMS has to look at her daughter, whose smile will put her sadness in perspective, and remind her that in a very real way we did achieve our dream. We created something precious, together, in the midst of very dark times.

Is that not what love is all about?

CHAPTER 5
Cancer cycle

Currently my life is cyclical. It fluctuates in a two-weekly pattern between well and unwell, between normality and nausea. In the well times, it is easy to pretend there is nothing wrong. It is easy to pretend that life continues as normal, with power bills and cooking. And then, just as normality feels as though it might last forever, it comes crashing to the ground with more chemo.

Chemo is a two-weekly ordeal for me this time around. It is the punctuation mark at the end of the normal week, just to emphasise that normality is not a given, but a privilege. Its fortnightly cycle comes around too soon to make you forget. But that is exactly what I wish I could do . . . forget.

I want to forget that I have cancer. I want to forget that death is running me down faster than it should be. I want to forget that I will be putting friends, family and Hannah through so much heartache. I want to forget that whatever suffering this world serves up is an indiscriminate force that chooses no one in particular, but is as arbitrary as the direction of the wind.

And then I feel well again, beginning to feel what life used to be like for me. Pretending that normality is the way my life is going, that I am well, that Hannah and I will have family . . .

Shattered by the next round of chemo . . .

Cyclical.

'I just want normality', The Boredom Blog, February 9, 2010

The cycles of my life, which over the past six years have been dominated by my treatment, have become smaller and smaller as I have approached the end of this particular road. Like a coiled spring being pulled ever tauter, the cyclical nature of my response to the ever-dominant spread of this disease throughout my body governs my weeks, my days, my hours. Even down to minutes.

There is what you might call a normal, or typical, daily routine. It is governed by sleeping and waking, my own and Elise's. She wakes early, and she is usually asleep again by the time I wake up. My 'waking up' is taking longer each day, so a whole morning full of activity can have occurred by the time I wake properly. Elise is up again in the afternoon, and that is when we play, though playtime is becoming harder as well. Friends will visit, sometimes late in the morning, sometimes around mid-afternoon. We have brought most of these visits to an end now. There are one or two goodbyes left to say over the next week or so, then they will be over, too.

Evenings are variable. Dinner, television, some more play-time between Elise and me. But, like most babies, Elise becomes grumpy in the evening, so 'play' is a little hit and miss.

Running parallel with this is the cycle of palliative care. With no particular goal in view, this cycle is about check-ups. It ensures my comfort and checks on infection, pain and levels of suffering. The components of this are daily, too—visits from the hospice staff, check-ups by the doctor, washes, pain relief, drainage checks. Some of these cycles are hourly, and will continue this way until the end, ever-reducing cycles of time until there is no space for time to exist. Then it all stops.

At the start, everything seemed to be on a yearly cycle, coin-ciding with the end of the academic year. Initial diagnosis, November 2008. First relapse and terminal diagnosis, November

2009. Graduation, November 2010. A bigger turn of the wheel then until the beginning of 2012, and the first real offer of hope—followed by an even more devastating pronouncement three months later. Second relapse, May 2012. Third relapse, November 2013. Death . . . October 2014.

And throughout that whole time, the difficult fortnightly cycle of chemotherapy. From the very beginning, a two-hour infusion of Oxaliplatin, two weeks of tablets twice a day, then a week off to recover before it all starts again. The treatment would later change to fortnightly infusions but otherwise generally follow the same pattern. Over and over again. For almost five full years. Eighty-nine rounds of it. Oncologists I have met reckon this must be some kind of record. It is a badge of honour I would prefer not to have been awarded.

All of that comes to this. There is a problem with the drainage tube that comes out of the right side of my abdomen. The suture has come undone, which means the tube could fall out. The question is, what do we do about it? Answer, probably nothing. The tube has been in there so long, a natural tunnel has formed out to the skin—a natural drain, so to speak. I discovered it just an hour ago. This, along with a number of other things, falls under the category of managing the day. That is what remains now. That is what life becomes. At the end.

———————

The events of our lives to which we attribute most significance more often than not happen innocuously, without fanfare or chorus, without angels appearing to herald what's about to take place, without commentary or flash cards or speech bubbles or announcements on the evening news. A sickness that results in death can begin with a niggle or a pain for which you can find a dozen different explanations other than the one that is responsible, the one that is so serious you never would have imagined it.

I had been plagued by stomach problems for two years, after a bout of Delhi belly on my trip to India the year that I met Hannah. It never settled down, at least back to what I considered normal, but I did not believe this was anything out of the ordinary. I self-diagnosed my upsets as post-infectious irritable bowel syndrome, which occurs often enough in people who have had such a terrible bout of food poisoning that the stomach and the gut lining take a couple of years to settle. That is what I assumed I had—nothing too serious, and not a major impact on my life, making me just slightly less tolerant of fatty and high lactose foods.

But here we were in November 2008. Almost a year on from our wedding, on the verge of big steps forward—our overseas trip culminating in hospital work in Africa, then a move to Rotorua. We were in Dunedin, sharing a pre-Christmas Christmas with Hannah's family, since we would not be around on the actual day. And that is when I started to get stomach-aches.

I figured it was something I had eaten the night before. The nature of the discomfort was odd, though. I had cramping pain that would last for 30 seconds to a minute, subside for twenty minutes, then come back again. I stopped eating to give my stomach a chance to recover, but rather than settling down the pain got worse. Over the next couple of days, the discomfort not only continued, it progressed. And by the time we had flown back to Auckland to prepare for our trip out of the country just three days later, my condition had worsened so much I realised I was going to need treatment. In the early hours of Wednesday I was vomiting. Lots of things cause progressive abdominal pain and vomiting—not least, appendicitis—but whatever it was, I would need to get it treated before we travelled. I sat in emergency for five hours; they were not really sure what the cause of the pain was when they admitted me for 'conservative observation', which essentially means they will not do much other than watch to see if it clears up or gets any worse. And I did get worse. Much worse. But on the chance it might be constipation they gave me a high-powered oral clearing fluid for my bowel. And that triggered what I remember as a very bad spell. I was very sick. My belly blew up like a beach ball. I needed a nasogastric tube. They did more X-rays, and the X-rays found air and fluid levels in my bowel and big dilated loops in the colon, which meant they now knew there was a blockage of some description. And I knew this before I went into surgery. I also knew that the most common cause of a bowel obstruction presenting with these symptoms was still appendicitis. I was 27. I had no risk factors for anything else. No family history. No associated symptoms suggesting it was anything more serious. I went into surgery knowing that it would be highly unusual for it to be anything else.

Surgery took place on the Friday night—the day we were due to fly out.

Let me share my reflections on the timing of this, based on the many hours of contemplation I have given it over the years. It could be viewed as cruelly ironic, the fact that on the very day Hannah and I were headed out on our big adventure I was, instead, having surgery. I knew by the time I was taken into theatre that we would have to cancel our trip. Or part of the trip, at least. If it was appendicitis we would still be able to pick up our plans after recovery. In hindsight, and setting aside the seriousness of what was actually going on, the timing of my sickness and subsequent operation could not have been better. Had I had a bowel obstruction in Nepal a week later there was a very good chance I would have suffered a perforated bowel and got sepsis and died. Had my illness presented just five days earlier, it would have disrupted my fifth-year exams, the most significant exams at med school. Much later, and it would have occurred in a Third World country. There is never a good time to get a partial bowel obstruction, but mine was timed with about as much clinical precision as was possible.

That is not to romanticise the seriousness of what happened or claim any particular divine influence, though it is part of the thread I have referred to already. The fact remains, I did not want to be in surgery on this or any other day, whether for appendicitis or anything else they might find.

I knew that a typical appendectomy takes 45 minutes to an hour to complete. My operation lasted three and a half hours, which I became aware of as I woke up in the post-anaesthetic care unit of Auckland City Hospital late at night. It is not a place where visitors are allowed, but since Hannah was a doctor working at the hospital, she was there at the bedside when I came to. My first question was whether it was appendicitis. She said no. For reasons I do not remember clearly, I asked if it was a neoplasm—this is medical jargon for cancer, best used only if your wife is a doctor. She said that she would rather the surgeon talk to me. I said no, I wanted her to tell me. And she said yes, they found a tumour that was obstructing my bowel. They performed what is called a right hemicolectomy—basically a removal of the right side of my bowel, the two remaining parts of which they then rejoined.

You cannot know, at that stage, what the tumour is. It could be benign. But as I woke up from the anaesthetic haze, the whole reality of what was happening began to sink in. What could this be? How serious was it? I knew that to have a tumour implied some kind of cancer, but I would not know what kind it was until the histology came back several days later.

We waited six days. And the histology confirmed that it was an adenocarcinoma of the bowel, its stage denominated T3N2M1, which means it was reasonably advanced—indeed, about as bad as it gets. Prognosis: a five-year survival rate of 40 per cent, less than a 50–50 chance of surviving beyond the five-year mark, which is the timeframe that represents a 'cure'. In other words, I had less chance of beating this than the odds riding on a coin toss.

It all hit home with this news.

For one thing, we would have to cancel our trip.

And yeah . . . I've got cancer.

I was discharged from hospital on my 28th birthday.

I remember a blog I posted about a year after this first diagnosis that took issue with people who said my life had taken a turn for the worse. I took issue on the basis that life is what it is, and that essentially life is more dynamic when we engage the peaks and the troughs and acknowledge the realities of our world, including its suffering, and incorporate all of our experiences into how we create meaning. My life took an unexpected detour, not a turn for the worse. And yet, I received news of my cancer like anyone would. Nobody likes being told they have cancer. Nobody. It just hits you. And there are tears. And there is fear. From the start, though, I resolved to be in the 40 per cent of people who make it. The odds were still in my favour—not greatly, but I had an almost 50–50 chance of not dying, of actually surviving. You could say it is a form of denial that you live in for a time, this belief that you could be one of the survivors, but you hold onto this hope for as long as you can—until they tell you there is no point holding onto the hope any longer.

After eight rounds of chemotherapy in that first year, we went on our South-East Asia trip. For all we knew, this first few months of chemo had knocked the cancer on the head. And I remember us walking around a lake in Vietnam, talking about what coming back to New Zealand was going to be like. We asked ourselves about what faced us on our return, and I remember crying, saying to Hannah, 'I don't want to die of this.' I was still in that 40 per cent bracket, but the thought of the realities we potentially confronted brought me face to face with all its attendant emotion.

I still feel the emotion of that day. It comes to me, unbidden. A moment in which there was still hope, a life-filled moment, a suspended reality. Dreams are still possible in such moments.

My life had not taken a turn for the worse. I still hold onto that. But I did not want to die. There was too much in life that I wanted to do. There was too much service I wanted to give to God. My emotion about this persisted for that whole first year of treatment, I realised later. Was it fear? Was it disappointment? Was it regret? I know that when the tears come now they are about lost opportunity. There was still so much yet to do.

I am covered in scars from my years of treatment. There is a hole in my side for my drain that is giving me trouble. There is an old scar up near my left clavicle that is the site of the second portacath through which they infused the chemo. There is another scar near my right clavicle where the first portacath was inserted. That one resulted in a thrombosis (blood clot) of the internal jugular vein, which meant a removal of the portacath and infusions of chemo via alternating arm veins. I have an intrathecal pump in my back for the pain relief in my abdomen. And there are great, long scars at the base of my stomach from the laparotomies they have carried out. Massive surgeries some of these, with recovery times of four to six weeks. My nightshirt falls open, revealing the scar on my abdomen. No chance that I can forget what the desire to survive has carved into my skin.

We returned from South-East Asia to a three-month follow-up scan, to determine how effective eight rounds of chemo had been. The scan revealed my first relapse.

Everything changed from this point, really. I could no longer live in the bittersweet denial of the 40 per cent. The cancer had spread to the paraaortic lymph nodes. Three nodes came back looking larger than normal. Regardless of where it was, the recurrence meant the cancer had not been discovered early enough. It could have recurred anywhere in the body. I could no longer speak of a chance of survival. When I asked the oncologist what it all meant, in terms of prognosis, he said we could no longer talk about five-year survivals—we talk now about two-year survivals. He never used the word 'terminal', but that is what he was saying. In other words, you will not survive this. This will kill you.

By virtue of the fact that they occur in young people in the first place, cancers in younger people are often aggressive. And this was certainly aggressive. This was a game changer, in all respects. This was no longer about cancelling a trip and claiming travel insurance, this was now a matter of life and death, and of deciding what I would focus on and hope to achieve, and how to pursue meaning and significance during my dying days. I had no idea how long I had—perhaps eighteen months, maybe the full two years—but there were no guarantees. It is still difficult for me to find words to describe how I actually felt. Emotionally, that is. I was never angry. I think I was frustrated. I definitely felt disappointment, probably more than anything else. You build up your life to be just the thing you want it to be, then it gets shattered in front of you. This was now five and a half years after the call to go to med school that changed my life, a reorientation that had led to marriage, brought me to the very cusp of qualifying to be a doctor, a dream I had harboured for ten years. And so, for me, it was just a sense of deep, deep sadness. Heartbreaking loss.

If you look over my blog posts from the period just after we received this news, there is a dramatic shift in their tone. They are given titles such as 'Life's not fair', 'Every moment', 'Beautiful . . . and ugly'. They become reflective and philosophical, seeking some sense of balance, of justice, of meaning. They are agonised and often agonising reflections on the harshest reality we face—that we die. We all die. Just not so young. And then there was Christmas, a time when such devastating news tends to hit home. I have already said how sickened I was by how commercial Christmas had become, particularly now that commercialism could not change what was wrong with me. Christmas this time around made me think very differently. Every time someone asked what I wanted for Christmas, I wanted to say, 'How about a cure for cancer?' What I realised was that everything someone might buy for me would have a longer lifespan than me. It was not more stuff that I needed. It was more life. It was the ability to not die.

Hannah heard the oncologist's news at my side, where she has always been. We came home together and talked the implications through between ourselves. That was okay. But then we had to ring our parents. And that is when the full weight of what we were facing hit us. It has been this way several times now over recent years. For the most part we have taken the bad news together, but there have been times when we have heard bad news alone. Telling one another has been hard enough, but getting on the phone and telling your parents, then your siblings . . . that is very tough. Each time, you face the emotion again. You relive your own grief and disappointment, hear their tears as your own and compound the sadness you already feel deep inside. I am thinking now of my mum, who as a nurse knew more than most the implications of what I was saying. I heard her crying on the end of the phone, then heard the family's tears as well. Mum would have found it as tough as Hannah and I have, because she was the one who went on to tell the rest of the family. She would have relived the grief over and over as we had.

The cancer is back and there are no survival chances this time. There is no easy way to say this to the people who love you and who have been praying that they would never hear these words. The sorrow is unbelievably difficult to face. But then life continues. It has to. And you literally do pick yourself up and start again. For me, that meant two things. The first was accepting that I was going back onto chemo. And this happened almost immediately. But this regime was different, and the impact on me not as severe. The regime of the previous months had taken me out for a good ten days at a time. Once I was up and running on the new regime, I discovered I was out for only five days, then had nine days of feeling well. On that basis, I figured I was up for continuing my studies, regardless of whether sickness or death would end them prematurely.

My calling to medicine was so strong at this point that it rallied me. I could not imagine doing anything else. I certainly would not be doing nothing. I had no hope of finishing my studies, and was almost certain that I would be too advanced in my sickness to graduate, but all I knew was that I felt this strong calling and that I had to keep going. I could not see it being any other way. So life started again. The goal of my treatment was to slow the growth of the cancer and perhaps even see a reduction. The outcome of this was a prolonged life for as long as the cancer was kept at bay. The key word was stability. A stable disease meant that I could perhaps be around beyond the following year. About a month or two after going back onto chemo, I approached the med school and outlined my situation. I could devote nine days out of every fortnight to my studies. I had to forego my elective and make up extra time, but I knew I could manage the workload in the times between my treatment. After considering my case, they approved my final year of study. Even so, I went back the following January genuinely thinking I would not finish.

I guess, in hindsight, I thought that if God had called me so strongly into medicine, then God was going to help me through it, so it was worth a shot. And I wanted to get back to it. That was the drive. It was my passion. I wanted to do what I loved. This is what got me through another twenty-odd rounds of chemo over that year, as well as the studies. I loved medicine. I still love medicine.

As it turned out, my body tolerated the chemo quite well. And it kept the cancer stable. It had grown millimetres between scans, well within the margins of error, and so we just kept going with the chemo. The cancer was tiny compared with what I have now. Even so, there was no way to know how it would continue to respond to treatment. Most die within the two years. Some die within three to six months. But we just kept going, notching up more and more rounds.

And I defied even my own expectations. Because I did not really believe I would graduate from med school, I had neglected to follow the typical pathway into a hospital position, which normally requires applications six months out from graduation. I had no idea where I would be in six months so did not put one in. I went to the hospital outside the normal process and explained the situation, as I had with med school. I asked them to employ me on the basis that I could guarantee nine days out of every fortnight for as long as the treatment continued to work. That was a two-thirds full-time commitment. And they said yes.

I graduated on November 15, 2010. My surgery to remove the tumour was on November 14, 2008. Two thousand and nine had been lost to chemo, but 2010 was my year—a year in which I learnt more about the power of a calling and how a conviction that is bigger than death can find meaning, purpose and fulfilment in the face of great sadness. I posted a blog in February 2010 about the cycle of cancer—my treatment, the good days and bad days, the spinning wheel of drugs, nausea, fatigue and moments of normality. I also wrote that I wanted more than normality, I wanted significance. I wrote that I wanted something that reached into the lives and hearts of those around me and made the world a better place. And I wrote that God's plans were bigger than any we could conceive of for ourselves.

Those plans got me through that year. The calling and the passion, the significance of the vision, and the love that had grown in me for medicine, gave me stability and drive despite all the bad news I had received—news as bad it gets. I had no idea how long I would live, but by the time of my graduation I had already surpassed my wildest imaginings. When my cancer continued to show excellent response to my treatment, it became clear that it was time to start thinking of the future. Career, house, family . . . who knew, perhaps even a cure! And a new voice. Suddenly doors opened up to share my story in ways I had never considered. The vision I had worked towards for so long might be over, but in spite of everything, a new one was forming.

I had discovered my 'bigger than normality'.

CHAPTER 6
Antihero

If we try to find our purpose in the ending, we only end up losing ourselves in the process of getting there. What I have discovered is that the purpose is in the journey, no matter where that journey leads us. The path we are on, no matter how successful or unsuccessful, is littered with stories of meaning, of relationships and of purpose. Through finding meaning in the journey, I am at peace that my outcome will *not* be the fairytale ending. I have found purpose in the day-to-day living of my life. The colours are brighter, the relationships more vivid, and what it means to serve humanity is more apparent. I'm okay with dying, and I have come to that place by finding meaning and purpose in the journey rather than the destination.

This is why I'm an antihero. I don't talk about conquering, overcoming or being the victor. I talk about the reality of suffering in my life and why I'm at peace with that. I talk about why, more often than not, there is no fairytale ending.

'The antihero', The Boredom Blog, January 15, 2011

Dying is a boring business. Nobody really tells you that. They tell you about the grim things that might happen to you along the way—the side effects of drugs and the pain and the anxiety—but no one ever tells you how boring it all gets. It is worse if you need to be around people, as I do. It used to be that if you put me in a room by myself for more than a day I would go crazy. I have not been by myself for four weeks, by any means, but the spells when there has been no one around and I have not had the energy to read or to write, or the cognitive functioning to do anything meaningful, down to texting or emailing or updating my blog, have been particularly hard. I am waiting, after all. That's the truth of it. Waiting for the body to surrender.

And I have never been particularly good at waiting.

I know better, though, because I have been here before. And I know from experience how moments of boredom can germinate and produce the type of fruit you never imagined you were capable of producing—proving that it had little to do with you all along. When my chemo first began, almost six years ago, I would spend a day in hospital then three weeks at home. Ten days of those three weeks were hopeless, then I would take the rest of the time to recover. And I was seriously bored. Lots of time to kill. Watching movies, watching television, but creating nothing. Moving nowhere. Aimless and hopeless, existing only to get well enough to endure the next round. But on a whim I thought, 'Why not post about this?' About what it was like to be bored while having chemo. To share random bits of information I found on the web while I lay there bored. I had no grand plan, no illusions of being a writer, certainly no expectation that anyone would read it outside of the people who knew me best. Had I thought it might achieve anything, I never would have given it the dumb title 'The Boredom Blog'.

And so I began, with a random post called 'The birth of something new', on January 26, 2009, just a few days out from completing my first round of chemo. Apart from titbits of information and interesting articles, I would also share updates from my chemo journey. It was easier than sending out a mass email, and if anyone was interested in knowing what stage my sickness was at, they could follow along. This was something Hannah and I processed on leaving the hospital the very first time. Who would we tell, and how much would we tell them? Is there a system for drawing up who needs to hear what, who would be offended, and how we should communicate? But this was too hard. I did not mind everyone knowing everything—or at least knowing where they could come if they wanted to know more. I had nothing to hide. I like to live my life in an open way that engages with people—live it 'out there', so to speak. So that is what I did. And that is what 'The Boredom Blog' became over that first year. Regular posts, sometimes several in a day in the early stage, featuring clippings, photos, medical updates full of esoteric terms most people would not understand without googling what they meant. I posted about a surprise trip to the Melbourne Grand Prix, tips for parenthood (in which I said I would not need these myself for about five to ten years), but mainly descriptions of the chemo and the effects it was having on my body.

But the blog's character changed when my life changed, several months later, with my first relapse and the knowledge that my time was now limited. In many ways, this was a more fundamental shift than the initial cancer diagnosis—probably because, as a pragmatic person with medical training, I could not avoid the sure knowledge that the recurrence meant the end. I posted an article titled 'Original intentions', flagging this shift. I alluded to the whimsical nature of the blog over the preceding months and said that while the updates on my condition would continue, the blog posts would now be less frequent, and more reflective and creative in nature. And you can feel the shift immediately. My posts became theological, self-reflective, melancholy. They were musings on life and death, suffering and hope, justice, meaning, value, purpose. I began to talk about faith more openly and was transparent about the impact that the things we take for granted—such as Christmas, or nature, or random moments of no apparent significance—were having on me now that I knew I was dying. It was a way of processing, too, of challenging myself to come up with words to describe the changes that were occurring in me. One post in those first few months post-relapse was titled 'Cancer and cynicism', and that was a rebuke to myself as well as others over the excuses we make to feel sorry for ourselves and to believe that we have it worse than anyone else. Cancer was the ultimate trump card, the ultimate conversation stopper, but I was being reminded constantly that injustices far more horrific than what I was experiencing are being perpetuated around the world, and the challenge for me was not to ask why I had suffered but what I could do to make a difference in the world. Even as a dying man.

So I stopped posting about the things that made me bored. But I was back at med school, too, and I had no excuse to be bored anymore. I had found my way back onto the path I was meant to be on, and all these converging elements—my medical studies; my determination to follow my calling despite my sickness; my very real suffering; and the psychological, spiritual and physical transformations I was experiencing—gave me fodder with which to write and to challenge myself, others, the status quo, the lazy conclusions we arrive at about life that give us comfort but are rarely based in reality.

Around this time I asked the followers of my blog whether I should change its name, given 'The Boredom Blog' was no longer apt. But it stuck. Nobody wanted it to change. And perhaps that was prophetic. Because here I am, still writing my reflections, about to die, and at times I am as bored as I was at the beginning.

The blog began with no sense of purpose, certainly with no expectation, hope or even suggestion that it would become something that might go some way to replacing the vision Hannah and I had lost. Perhaps that is why, when opportunities for my story to be heard began to come, and the emergence of a new role began to take shape, it was not as someone who had achieved or overcome great adversity or experienced miraculous healing. It was really just about being me, just a guy being honest about his own wrestle with the sometimes-brutal realities we all face at one time or another.

_____

While all this was going on in my private world—the developments in my health, and my marriage, and my vocation—there was the parallel journey of my faith community. Because of the cancer, Hannah and I did not move to Rotorua, so we stayed connected with the community we had helped to start. Its members had become some of our closest friends and stood beside us as we processed the shock of the initial diagnosis, then the relapse. I mention the community here because their work was not only running parallel to the work I would soon be invited to pursue, but their ideas of community were very much tied to the passion I continued to have for people and for reaching people in the place of their own struggles. We shared a particular view of what community was—not a static, closed club, but a movement that is constantly pushing outwards beyond itself, a dynamic and organic movement whose energy is always radiating outwards in a gesture of embrace. In my understanding of community, it is constantly expanding outwards through space and time to reach others. And this fuelled my passion for what emerged because of the blog, and because of my story and my willingness just to admit that we live in a broken world where crap is part of our daily routine. I was aware that very often in the West, we are immune from a lot of that crap, and we forget—or we deny—that it happens. And when it happens to us? We cry foul. Shit happens in this life and we just get all moody when it happens to us instead of others. No amount of faith was necessarily going to alter that fact. It was up to us to strive for significance in the face of that. I believed that others wanted and needed to hear this message, and this proved to be the case.

But what was ultimately going on was a rediscovery of my own longstanding sense of purpose and significance. I was finding this back at med school and I would ultimately find it in my work. I was also finding it at home, in our marriage and in my involvement with the community. But my vision had been a global one, of making a difference overseas. This added value to my work, in a way, and this is what I had lost. But I was rediscovering it again through the blog and the opportunities to share my story that came with it. I was also discovering that this question of purpose and meaning, and value beyond consumerism and selfish ambition, was a question many people my age and younger were distressed about. I encountered many young people who were wondering what their lives were all about and what it was they were trying to achieve. The question was being raised by both people of faith and people without faith—the only difference between them was the language they used to express it. I became unsure about whether people needed a calling in their life at all. I discovered that so many people were hung up about it—perhaps all they needed was to know that they were just free to live, without worrying about any great purpose or grand design. I felt that I was fortunate in that I did have a clear direction, but I was not, and am not, convinced that everyone needs or has one. People do not always see the significance of their lives or their jobs or their relationships in a bigger picture. It does not mean the bigger picture is not there. Not everyone gets to see the impact they are having on the world.

It took some time for Hannah and me to make the adjustments we needed to default back to the community we had been part of, and also to forge a new path. This was a mental adjustment as much as anything else. It was not long before we appreciated the value of what we were pursuing in place of the dreams we had had. And many of the directions I took in my speaking and media work began as a direct result of the relationships we had formed before my diagnosis. A friend in our faith community was the director of the biggest Eastercamp in New Zealand, so before too long, I was up in front of 5000 kids, telling them that I was dying and why that was okay.

———————

My idea of greatness had always revolved around achieving significant change in the world, most likely on the back of my medical work. My idea of service was aligned with this. I would work on behalf of others, and strive to make as much of a difference in the lives of people as I could with the time, skills and resources I had. In med school before Diagnosis Day I had considered moving into specific specialties largely because of the exponential impact those specialties might produce in certain contexts around the globe. Ophthalmology was one area, because on very little money and with a relatively minor surgical procedure (on cataracts) you can have a massive impact, often on entire communities. In helping people return to work you not only help them and their families, you influence the economy of an entire community. My whole adult life, I have carried inside me what I have called a rage, a conviction about inequality and injustice, and the desire not only to make a difference as a doctor but also to challenge frameworks of corruption and inequality. It was never my intention to be a 'hero' in the classical sense, but in my conviction that I was being called to 'greatness' I never imagined that I would achieve anything from a position of vulnerability and weakness. The opposite, in fact.

But this is precisely what began to emerge. I was invited to tell my story at a Promise Keepers NZ event in Auckland. Promise Keepers is an international organisation for men that holds conventions and rallies to get men thinking about issues they face and how faith might help them engage with those issues. My story of vulnerability, and of my goals essentially having been taken away, is not one that men typically find encouraging. Despite this, the event went very well, and I was invited to take a more prominent role in other rallies being held around the country. After the event, an acquaintance who works in the media verbalised what I was suspecting—I was not a typical hero of the Christian faith. He said that people were not celebrating my response to some great and glorious miraculous healing, but my response to what was going to be my ultimate end. I had none of the criteria of the typical hero of the faith. I was the opposite. And yet, I was being called a hero for that. I was a contradiction.

He was the first to use the term 'antihero' to give narrative shape to my message. The antihero is an atypical figure. If you consider the generic narrative of the heroic journey, it tells the tale of a protagonist who sets out on a quest and encounters a great obstacle. In overcoming that obstacle the hero's character is revealed and the story finds resolution. I was never going to overcome my obstacle. It was going to overcome me. But what seemed to connect with audiences at these events was the story of someone who, while accepting that he was facing his demise and would not be miraculously healed (though I still prayed for this), had not given up on his faith or his calling or his passion to make a difference. I came to realise that my story was not normally held up as one to emulate in our society and in our time, where the heroes we look to are people of superhuman strength and courage. I was not a superhero. I was going to be destroyed, and not even by something as exotic as kryptonite. But somehow, my story touched a nerve, and despite everything, the audiences, from adult men to teenage boys and girls, found it encouraging.

This happened by accident and was a surprise to me as much as anyone. For me, it was just the reality of my situation, not a story I had made up to bring people to faith or to encourage people whose faith was faltering. It was just my life and it still is. The reality is that I am now in the penultimate stage of that story, the antihero's tale. For me, it is not an uplifting testimony or a paradigmatic narrative. It is a hard, sorrowful and all-too-slow demise. It is actual life and death. I will actually die. I will actually be overcome.

And just to bring the ironic subtext into the foreground—I have become the person I wanted to help. That is how flipped around my story has become. When I envisaged myself as the hero in a story in which entire communities of underprivileged and suffering people would be impacted by my work, what I actually saw were people who are in the position I am in now. I have become them, the people I was meant to serve. There is nothing heroic in that.

There would be one more chance at becoming the hero before my number was called. And that would emerge in the early part of 2012—a carrot, offering Hannah and me hope, and me the opportunity to take off the mantle of the antihero and become a more traditional hero, more like the character I had in my mind. But it was not to be. I was doomed to play this particular role to the very end.

The role of the antihero is not one for which people volunteer. When they get kids to put up their hands for parts in the school play, no one is jumping for the chance to play the antihero—if there even is an antihero in the story. And it was not one that I assigned to myself, either. I take no credit nor deserve any for the role I came to play in this particular drama. In fact, I remember those first few days after my first relapse, after having been told that my disease was terminal. In a strange way, you are suddenly thrust into the spotlight when you least want to be. That first evening, my parents came around just to hang out— just to be near us. This was the immediate response of others, too. When we told our concentric rings of family and friends, we found that others wanted to come over and be around us. But you sit there in sadness. A moroseness comes over the room, a melancholy for which you know you are responsible. And it is acutely obvious to everyone there that you are only hanging out because you have just been told you are going to die. Suddenly, you are the central character in a story you do not want to be in. You are the centre of attention, the person everyone is talking about. It is a focus you do not want, but you are in the starring role and there is no way out. It is not like school, where you can wag a day and get out of the play. There is no contract to tear up. You are in this role because a disease inside you cannot be stopped. The inevitability of the outcome, the glare of the spotlight, the volume of the voices speaking your name, and the weight of the gloom that has settled like ash over everything because of you and this disease you are carrying . . . who would opt for this part?

When I talk about going through the last door first—that door marked 'Trust and Submission'—it was here that it was presented to me as my only hope. What else could I do in the face of these realities but go to the God of my faith tradition, the faith I had made my own, and say, 'Okay, I trust you, and in trusting I will go wherever that path leads me'? I resolved then and there to say yes to any opportunity that came my way, to throw myself into life with a fervour that many cancer sufferers experience, but also to follow the peculiar paths I could not yet foresee. And of course, by making that statement, things escalated to a level that only now, in reflection, can I recognise as a direct consequence of walking through that door.

At some point there was a shift, an awakening to the knowledge that this was now my work—a different type of calling to the one I had previously, but perhaps not so far removed. I saw what I was doing as part of the bigger picture I had been pursuing passionately all along, the pragmatic outworking of faith in ways that made the world a better place—the propagation of peace, addressing poverty and ill-health, righting injustices—what some people of faith call 'kingdom work'. This idea was important to me, and always had been. And there was definitely a growing awareness in me that while I was not doing what I had originally envisaged, I was at least contributing something. I did not set out thinking I was going to help people work through their sickness or challenge and encourage their faith—nothing like that. But as readers of the blog or people who heard me tell my story responded with feedback about how they had been helped and how much my story was impacting people, it motivated me to keep going. I did not know at that stage why it was helping people—I just accepted that it was. And this gave me a greater sense of purpose and a determination to keep telling my story.

I was writing for myself. The things I reflected on were struggles I was having, thoughts I was processing. But, for whatever reason, what I put out there in the blogosphere took on a life of its own and went far beyond what it was intended to be.

I have had some dark days in recent weeks. At the most despairing times, when I have been overwhelmed by some of the symptoms associated with dying, I have thought about what it is that keeps me holding on. One thing that holds it together for me even now is the accountability of the antihero to the people he has influenced with his story. The antihero holds out to the end, does not give up, does not lose faith. And I mean to the very end—no matter what happens in coming days. The antihero does not get two days out from death and suddenly proclaim he got it all wrong. He somehow finds strength in weakness, right to the last.

Six months on from my terminal diagnosis I got my first invitation to tell my story, at a church Hannah and I had been involved in before we were married. The message I put together was the same message I gave on multiple occasions to different people at varying events over the following few years. The key points were my circumstances, my diagnosis and how I was dealing with it all. It has been refined over the years, but the core message is the same. It is my story, basically, no frills or embellishments, just my story. Over the last year I have spoken in public perhaps three times. But at the peak, I had a speaking engagement most weekends.

Those engagements included bigger events like Promise Keepers. That one event led to invitations to speak at subsequent Promise Keeper meetings in Dunedin, Christchurch and Tauranga. There were 2500 men at the Auckland event. I have spoken at the Parachute Music Festival in Hamilton. I have also been to each of the Eastercamps since my diagnosis, including the last one, mainly to be camp doctor (with Hannah and Elise) but also, at times, to speak. Up to 5000 kids attend that camp. The first year I spoke, I was backstage after my talk when someone told me to check out what was happening in the auditorium. I looked out and saw 1200 kids up out of their seats and wandering down to the stage area at the front, responding to an invitation to come forward for help or advice, or to share stories or get counsel, or to talk about faith. To see my story affect so many at one time was humbling. I only have my simplistic language of faith to make sense of what was stirring in the room in that moment.

The more I told my story, the more people heard it, and the more people heard it, the more invitations I received—not to tell a different story, but to tell the story they had heard already, but in a different forum. It was the story of the antihero they wanted. That story was a thumbnail sketch of the life I have reflected on over these past few weeks, the glimpse I hope to leave behind for Elise. In the twenty-minute version I talked about the life I thought I had and the path I thought I was following. I was certain I had been called to go in a particular direction, but then it all fell apart. I talked about the diagnosis and the chemo and everything that had happened since. As the story continued in real time, so the story I was telling developed. There were more disappointments, and more seasons of hope. My life for the past six years has had its own episodic dramas, its own narrative arc. It has been a tale of highs and lows, of moments of belief followed by moments of despair. Whenever I thought there was a chance of things resolving and providing that miracle moment we were praying for, those thoughts were abruptly shattered by bad news. And there were remarkable moments of life in there, too, all of which I incorporated into the telling. I drew on some stories from the New Testament as well—Jesus in the Garden of Gethsemane the night before his execution, for example. I talked about the two halves of his prayer, the one half we pray well ('Take this suffering away'), the other half not so well ('but I trust God anyway'). His is such a human story—honesty followed by submission—and I have always used it as the blueprint for my own struggle. My prayer has always been: 'I do not want to die, but if I have to, I will accept that.'

There is another story I use, of a blind man who goes to Jesus for healing. The point of the story is not the healing itself, but the response of the disciples who are following Jesus, who ask why the man was born blind. They want a good theological answer that makes sense of his suffering. The futility of that why question has stuck with me over the years and became a key part of my story. I realised early on how futile the question 'Why?' was. There are no answers—and even if there were, what could we do with them? But the fact that even in our weakest moments we can choose to find meaning and value, and essentially keep our focus on what we do for others—that, to me, was the real story. And that was what happened with the blind man. It was not about the reason why—it was about the what next?

The human instinct is to ask why. Why do I have cancer? Why has my spouse just died? Why has my business failed? Why was I fired? More often than not, no answer presents itself, but it is the motivation behind the question that remains unfulfilled. Our intention is actually to blame or to seek restitution, or perhaps even to change our circumstances. And when this does not happen—because it cannot happen—we become despondent and disillusioned. And then we ask more why questions. And we spiral down into ever more disappointing realms of uncertainty about, and dissatisfaction with, life—all the while missing opportunities that presented themselves to contribute something unique and worthwhile to the human endeavour.

So, the question is not 'Why?' but 'How?' How can I create something in the context of this terrible situation? How can I serve someone despite my own suffering? How can I make a difference to someone else's life even though mine is about to run its course? In my experience, it is by asking these how questions that the opportunities have come. Had they come while I was focused on why questions, I would have missed them. They would have been anathema to me. It is impossible to recognise opportunities to help others or to build them up when you are caught in your own pity spiral, but I remember one guy—not a blind man, but a recovering alcoholic. He came forward at the Eastercamp after my talk. He said he had been an alcoholic his whole life but had been one year sober. He had been asking why for years—but after hearing my story he would ask how—how could he be used as an ex-alcoholic to help other alcoholics? In a way, he had been blind. Now he could see. And I was seeing too—seeing how my own weakness was empowering other people towards significant change.

The media opportunities followed. The first was a radio interview through a colleague at med school. That led to more radio.

Then a girl tracked me down through the blog for a current affairs story that would appear on New Zealand television. She was 30 years old, had been diagnosed with the same cancer as me, and had founded a group called Beat Bowel Cancer Aotearoa. It was a patient- and family-initiated group pushing for legislative change to speed up the advancement of bowel cancer treatment in New Zealand, since we fall way behind the global standards. Of course, I happily gave them my support.

The story appeared on a current affairs program called *20/20*, and featured both of us together. Unfortunately, Claire died just six weeks after the story aired. A year or so later, the *20/20* team came back to me for a follow-up. I suspected it was prompted by surprise that I was still alive. This time, they focused on my role as a doctor, as well as the story of my ongoing battle. When they heard that Hannah was pregnant, they made contact to do a further follow-up. And that quick follow-up escalated into a full story once Elise was born. Elise was in the media glare before she knew anything about it, something that prompted us to think about boundaries regarding how much exposure she had. But the people from the *20/20* team were genuinely thrilled to see something so wonderful come from something so terrible. And their joy was our thrill to witness. The mutual happiness that occurred around Elise's birth has provided many people with a rare moment of true gratitude in the context of what in other respects has been a tragic story.

Along the way, there have been other television appearances. There was a segment called 'Inspiring New Zealander of the Year', and other slots representing Beat Bowel Cancer Aotearoa, which had asked me to be an ambassador. But the biggest exposure by far was when I faced the very real prospect of dying before Elise was born. That took the story to levels we never could have foreseen.

Despite all of this, and precisely because I am a pragmatist and also someone who has remained committed to owning the reality of what he faces, as well as the faith that has shaped his convictions, I have to acknowledge the unresolved nature of my original calling. The question that hangs over the vision I was given, which I am as convinced of today as I was when it occurred, has not been answered. It is not a why question, which is the reason I can be at peace about the lack of resolution, but it is something that remains a mystery to me. You might say that I am content to sit with the tension of the peace I feel, juxtaposed with the unanswered aspects of what did not eventuate. It takes some people 90 years to fully understand key moments in their life, to have access to ideas and thoughts that give them a framework of understanding, ideas that may not have been available to them when those moments first happened. I do not have 90 years. I do not have 90 days. I am running out of time to have the type of insight I need to resolve this particular mystery, which is why I have to let go and accept that I am likely to die while I am still in the dark. I am amazed at the reach my story has had, and the media coverage it attracted, but I can also say that my role as antihero has been a consolation prize. Life would have been very different had I had my way. And in the face of this, all I can do is accept my circumstances and seek to make the best of them.

That is not to diminish what I have achieved or the people I have challenged and encouraged. I have not given this role half-measures. It has not been any less of a journey or produced anything less significant than the one I had imagined. Some would argue that in the short space of time it has occurred, it has been far more productive than my other path may have been. In some ways, it has been more fruitful than a career in medicine in the Third World might have become.

In any case, the antihero does not complain. The whole purpose of the role is to face what is, not get caught up in what should or might have been. More than anything, this has been a season of grace, with rewards and experiences I never would have scripted. My way would have looked quite different. But am I satisfied? Is that the word I would use, two weeks out from dying and looking back over this extraordinary time?

No. I am not satisfied.

But am I fulfilled?

Yes. I will die fulfilled, knowing I gave the last six years everything I had.

CHAPTER 7
More and more of life

It was in the context of gestating new life that I pursued more of my own life.

My daughter is literally the reason I am still alive . . .

And I will be forever grateful to her, and to those who enabled this to happen.

We now move forward into a new phase of life, one that will no doubt include sleepless nights, but filled with tears of joy and an overwhelming sense of pride in who our daughter has already become.

'Elise Alexandra Grace', The Boredom Blog, January 25, 2014

Two weeks ago we celebrated Father's Day. And Elise gave me presents.

I got some lollies, a model aeroplane and a few cards. What else? A ring, which is spinning around my finger. I now have a ring from each of my girls. And a book: *My Dad's the Coolest*. Because her dad *is* the coolest.

I found it tough buying presents for Hannah on Mother's Day. It must have been tougher to know what to buy for me. What do you buy the dad who is on his deathbed? Something sentimental, perhaps. Or something consumable.

Elise.

I simply do not have the words to convey the significance of that day. It was emotional, of course. There is hardly anything more sentimental than celebrating a significant day for the one and only time—and Father's Day at that. I was not meant to make it to Elise's birth, let alone to Father's Day, a whole eight months later. But its significance goes beyond the sentimental, in my mind anyway. It goes back before Elise was born, to some of the most hope-filled days her mum and I have experienced in this long and difficult journey. It goes back to a dream, if I am honest, and a walk around Cornwall Park, where we allowed ourselves just a moment to consider . . . what if? It was not a fanciful dream, or so we thought at the time. We had every reason at that moment to think that the unthinkable was within our reach. Every reason. It is an impossible situation, knowing in the back of your mind that you should keep the hope in balance, but feeling it rise ever more powerfully in your chest as you picture . . . no, taste, a life of not one, but two, three, five, ten more years. And if ten years, why not 50?

Then, almost two years to the day later, Elise was here, the most tangible manifestation of hope there could be—a living person, our child, born out of love, out of life, out of a dream.

For eight months, I have watched her grow. Enjoyed the way she has learnt to control her fingers, the intelligence in her eyes, her laughter, the way she communicates, her love of stories. I was away in hospital, then the hospice, for a short period, and in that time she grew so much. We had it so good for a while. Six months of relative normality was not bad, considering the shape I was in and the medication I had taken over the years. It was a blow to us all when I got sick again, because with the three of us in the home I had begun to dream. You could say I got lazy. I started to forget that I was dying. I know Elise will understand. She may not remember, but she will understand. We shared life for just a fleeting moment. And it was very, very good.

I want so much for Elise. Is Secretary-General of the United Nations too lofty a goal? I do not think so. Okay, perhaps I am joking, but just a little. I do believe, though, that she will have an extraordinary life. Even now I see that, when Elise is here on the bed with Hannah. I think she will make a difference, and on a big scale. On a global scale. The world will be her stage. Because I think that is what the world needs. The world needs Elise. I do not know how she will get there, or what the steps will be, but I know that God will walk beside her. That is her legacy.

Here is my hope. I hope that God's plans for Elise are bigger and bolder than the plans he had for me. I know it will be the case. How? Because I was there when she took shape in our dreams and when we fought to conceive and when we begged for time so that I could be there at her birth. So extraordinary, all of it. Supernatural, I would say, looking back.

And Elise is extraordinary already. So I already know. In her own way, Elise will make a difference in the world.

Towards the end of 2011, the game had changed, significantly. And very surprisingly. I had a CT scan in November that revealed almost zero advancement in my cancer, apart from a tiny amount of growth in the largest of the three nodes that were the focus of my treatment. My oncologist delivered the results with an accompanying explanatory narrative that it had clearly surprised him as much as it was about to surprise me. Essentially, my cancer was not behaving as it should. According to best estimates, I stood about a 20 per cent chance of lasting another year, but my cancer was not behaving as if it was playing by those odds. And with my lack of family history and the different ways my cancer had presented, the oncology team concluded they were dealing with a type of cancer they had not dealt with before. All cancers are different, and every cancer reacts in unique ways in every person and with every body in which it is growing. The characteristics of my cancer were very peculiar, placing it very much on the abnormal end of the spectrum. The long and short of this was that perhaps I was not one of the 20 per cent. Perhaps there were options that could prolong my life by treating the cancer in different ways. If the cancer was atypical, perhaps it needed an atypical response.

It does not take much imagination to picture the types of conversations that were happening behind the scenes. Specialists from multiple fields colluded to come up with a number of options. My cancer nodes were in troublesome places in my body, so several experts were having their say on how successful different options might be, and what complications might come along with them. But imagine what was going through my mind, and through Hannah's. Did we dare hope?

When I saw the oncologist again just a week later, I was presented with a lifeline, the first in a long time. This was a full two years after my terminal diagnosis, a full year after my graduation. It came after a year of working in the hospital. I was meant to be dead already. The two years I had been given to hope for, according to the statistics, were up, which was why my chances of living for a further twelve months were dropping. And this was no casual offer of life. It would involve major surgery—what is called a retroperitoneal lymph node dissection, requiring input from some of the top surgeons in the country. Apart from the normal risks associated with an operation, because of the location of the cancerous nodes I could lose a kidney and potentially become paralysed. Those chances were slim, but they were present. It was a lot to weigh up, but also not really. There were three potential outcomes from this course of action. The first was that the cancer would relapse, but faster and more aggressively. This meant that I would die sooner. But I was dying anyway, so this really did not change anything. The second outcome—there would be medium-term remission with no cancer for five to ten years, followed by a likely return of the cancer. Again, back to where we started, but with another five to ten years of life. The third option—and a possibility that had not been raised for several years—long-term remission, which meant I could potentially live another 50 years, dying of something else perhaps, or even the return of cancer from all the CT scans I'd had over the years.

It was a genuine offer of life—the gift of healing we had prayed for, dreamt of, never thought possible. Was it occurring to me also that this was how my vision would be reconciled with my reality? Was it going to be possible to resurrect yet another dream I thought was gone for good? I cannot remember how much attention I gave these thoughts, but it was like being placed back on the donkey. And in front of the donkey, tempting it along a brand new path, was a very large carrot.

I had the surgery on February 14, 2012, followed by a lengthy period of recovery, ten days of which I spent in hospital, followed by recuperation at home. Over the next month or so, my doctors talked more about how to give my body the best possible chance of beating cancer. The surgery had been a success. All the nodes had been removed and I emerged from theatre without having suffered anything more than the typical traumas to my organs during the procedure itself. By April, it had been decided to give me a course of radiation treatment. This was precautionary more than anything, but given the nature of my cancer and the options we had taken, it made sense. Potentially, chemotherapy was over. I had clocked up 41 rounds at this stage, which was a record even then, as far as we knew. And my goal of getting back to work by the end of May was still realistic.

Anyone in remission from cancer will agree that this period of not really knowing is almost as scary as the cancer itself. The fear of relapse is profound. Your life feels so fragile—the healthy state you have been granted is so precarious. You just do not know . . . if, when, how long? And, as with most things we do not know or understand, we fill the void with fear. We could be fine for two years, five years, ten or fifteen. But what if it comes back? This was not what I was thinking at the time, though. I remember feeling guilty, actually, to a degree. It was dawning on me more with each incremental step towards an inconceivable recovery that I actually might have a chance to live, and this was making me feel a range of different and conflicting emotions. I had just finished reading a book by someone who had become a friend of mine, Kristian Anderson, who, like me, had blogged about his battle with bowel cancer and who had died in January 2012, just three months earlier. I remember feeling guilty that I might live when he had died, because Kristian had children and I did not. Not yet. I would gladly have changed places with him, given him this lifeline I had been handed. Not for the first time, it made me confront the lack of fairness in life.

But . . . it turned out not to be a lifeline after all. I had not been granted another shot at life. The carrot being dangled in front of the donkey was snatched away, just as abruptly as the hope had been offered.

On May 16, I attended an outpatient appointment with the radiation oncologist to plan my therapy. There was no reason for me to be concerned about this appointment, which is why I was there alone. It was a routine oncology appointment. I'd had hundreds of them. I'd also had a scan the week before in preparation for the radiotherapy, so there was really no reason for me to expect bad news. The purpose was to map out the next phase of treatment, but bad news feels all the worse when you are not prepared for it, still swimming in the euphoria of possibilities. And that euphoria was short-lived, as it turned out.

The clinician turned up, sat down, and said to me casually, 'Oh, you've seen your results, right?' I said no. And he said, 'Oh.'

The news I did not, in all honesty, expect: the cancer was back, and aggressively so. A big lesion had been discovered in my liver (where it had never been before), and in other areas, too. This was about as bad an outcome as we could have had. I remember absorbing the news as a typical clinician—in that moment anyway. Perhaps the professional self kicks in at such times to keep emotion at bay, because I felt no emotion, just shock. This was a serious advance compared to any previous news I had received. It was almost too much to process. And I felt very alone.

The emotion came later. I went home and cried. I knew that telling Hannah would be harder than hearing the news myself. She was at work, at a clinic, learning stuff for her paediatric exams that were just three weeks away. I remember texting her, asking her to cancel everything she had on that afternoon and to come home. I tried to give her the news in writing, but could not. I would have to do it face to face. She would know from the text, though, that something was terribly wrong. She later told me that when she saw the number of missed calls on her phone, she thought someone close to us had died, so far from our radar was a cancer relapse.

The dream was shattered. That was the truth of it. I remember thinking how mean cancer was. It never spares your feelings. It does not play by the script and follow a path towards hope. This was harder to take than anything I had confronted before, because it came after our hopes had been built up so high. Now I knew for certain that cancer was going to get me. I was living on borrowed time.

My ideas about hope changed that day. I realised then and there that people place their hope in the wrong things. My hope had been in humanity's ability to address the issue of my life and death, to fix my problem. And in this case, humanity's ability was found wanting. I literally had to live with—and die with— the end of our dreams. Because in the context of hope, we had started to plan for the future. We could not avoid it. We began with family and planning for a child. We dreamt about what we could do with our lives now that there was a future. We dared. Dared to reformulate our vision. I was so convinced that this hope was tangible, I was feeling survivor's guilt. Survivor's guilt!

Hannah came home and we collapsed into each other's arms. I was right—she had been able to tell that something was very wrong. So we cried. Just held each other and cried, as we have at all the key moments.

This second relapse is a hinge point in my story, which is why it keeps coming back to me now. The hope was there, the dreams resurfaced, and the cruel reality of cancer hit me harder than before. Up until this point, I guess there was always something in the back of my mind that kept suggesting that maybe, just maybe, I could battle—and beat—this thing. It was my old competitive streak surfacing again. Tell me I have a 40 per cent chance, I will be one of the 40. Tell me it is 20 per cent . . . well, let's see about that.

But from this point on, May 2012, the fight I had in me to beat cancer ended. I accepted defeat. Cancer was going to kill me. I did not know when any more than I had before. It had recurred aggressively, but I would continue as I always had—on more chemo, this time with the goal of slowing the cancer that was now in my liver, my mesentery, and the lymph chain where they had operated. Who knew how long that would give me and what I could achieve in that time?

Was I angry? No. Was I despairing? I was disappointed. More than I can say. Gutted. Absolutely. But angry? I went back through that last door again, and just had to trust. Give up all that I was feeling and just trust in the bigger picture. Submit to the knowledge that bigger things are going on that I cannot influence or control. Perhaps this was supernatural, this trust. It feels so now, looking back. Thinking over those times from this perspective, I do not know how we got through and just kept picking ourselves up and starting again. At the time it did not feel supernatural. We just felt broken. And so, so vulnerable.

———————

Elise emerged in our conversations and in our dreams in the midst of all this. We began to think of a family before the bad news came, in that window of opportunity and hope. It was like an umbrella, that hope, shielding us from the storm we had faced for so long. We sheltered beneath it and gave ourselves the freedom to imagine a time when there would be no storm at all. And so we strolled through the park, dreaming, and Hannah said, 'What about children? Do you want to try to have children?'

Hannah was serious. And why not? Our friends were having kids. Hannah was not getting any younger, as they say. In a cancer-free world, children would have been on the agenda by now. Hannah probably had stronger feelings about it than I did, of course—I was still coming to terms with what a cancer-free world might allow us to achieve—but the seeds were planted, right there in a moment I have never forgotten. It was a lighter world in that brief period of time. The umbrella kept us sheltered, and we thought it would keep us safe, but then the bad news hit us and it was as if the storm had just snatched the umbrella from our hands and was blowing full into our faces. And yes, it was like mourning. It was like being diagnosed for the first time, but worse. Because the first time around we never fully realised the diagnosis meant that we would lose everything. This time there was no denying it. Even so, and even in the face of such a blow, the seeds of new life were already sprouting. We talked about the possibility of family again. Should we try anyway? What did we have to lose?

But there are only so many risks you can take at once. What if the disease could not be stabilised this time? What if it was more rampant and more aggressive than before? And so we waited. Waited to see how the year would go. But Elise was there, in our minds. And something else, too. The dream of family had given us hope and had given us life—despite what had happened. In the midst of that awful time, and in the face of such disheartening news, Elise gave us a future to hold onto. She helped us carry on. And somehow, that fired in me a great desire. To pursue my career, for one thing, and to pursue it as if I were not sick at all. To buy a house, too, and to be ready for when our family began. And to travel—to see places and taste food we had never experienced before. It is hard to believe now how focused we became on living. But that is what happens when you come face to face with your own mortality: you discover just how much you want to live.

So we waited, but we also moved forward. I made the first steps towards becoming a registrar, knowing full well that it might be utterly futile because of the clock that was keeping time on my life. I began chemo again, ticking off rounds 42, 43, 44. At work, I went back down to the two-thirds employment status that had been in place before my surgery. I had enjoyed being off chemo for six months, and in the final few weeks before chemo started up again I was beginning to feel like I did years earlier, before chemo had begun—it had taken almost all of six months to feel normal again! But it took just one weekend of chemo to remember what it was like. A weekend of life lost. A close encounter with nausea and vomiting. A reminder that I was mortal. If this regime failed, I was told, one remaining option would be Bevacizumab (Avastin), a non-funded drug in New Zealand that would cost $6000 for every fortnightly round, a total of $60,000 for a treatment that would give me maybe an increased life expectancy of three months—if that! I could not justify that sort of money for such a meagre result, not when the money could be spent on something like vaccines in the developing world— where each dollar spent would have a far greater impact. My outcome was inevitable and we were just delaying it. That money spent in a different context could change lives far more substantially, so there was little chance that I would be opting for Avastin.

There were no guarantees with any of the steps we were taking, and there was perhaps more uncertainty now than before surgery. But it did not seem to matter. We would just keep moving forward. I knew that just because my cancer had responded to chemotherapy before was no guarantee that it would do so again. The future was uncertain once more, and this tested my resolve. I blogged at the time that all human and natural sources of resolve were finite, ultimately. Eventually, exhaustion takes over. And that is what I am experiencing now. Back then, though, I knew I had some fight remaining in me and I was trusting in something bigger than me, constantly.

My first scan after going back on chemo showed that my disease had stabilised, yet again, and with the buoyancy that this news gave us we took some giant steps towards normality. By September we had bought our home—this house, where I am now, the home Elise was born into. We went to Italy that same month, and discovered places we would quite happily have returned to throughout our life together. On our return to New Zealand we moved house, and I got back to the business of treating cancer. But the dream about family did not die. It was very much alive. The devastation of the relapse had stolen so many of our dreams, as cancer had from the start, but this was one dream I wanted to see realised for Hannah's sake. And with a stable disease, our own home, and a determination to advance my career for as long as I could, it was time to start this new phase of the journey.

In late 2012, we made the first serious enquiries about the possibilities of having a family. For us, children meant in-vitro fertilisation (IVF). Chemotherapy destroys your sperm, or renders what sperm you have left quite questionable, in terms of genetic viability. I had sperm stored from before my treatment began, and we could leapfrog the usual waiting time because we had met with them some time before to consider our options when it came to fertility—and time was clearly of the essence, in my case at least. After considering everything carefully, we sat down with both sets of parents to gauge their support. We knew we could not take this step without their help. Our child would have higher needs than many. His or her father would not be around for long, which would necessitate more help from grandparents than a child born in 'ideal' circumstances. On Hannah's side of the family there were no grandchildren at the time. On my side, our child would be the fourth. But of course, both sets of parents were completely in support. In the case of my parents, it was like the restoration of one of their dreams, as well as ours. The idea that we might have kids one day was something they had written off completely.

By the end of the year, the first IVF cycle was underway. Yet again, we had allowed ourselves to hope, with no guarantees that anything would work. The initial egg transfer in November was unsuccessful. We had the Christmas break and then tried again. Another fail. We had three successful embryos from the first harvest, each of which failed. Typically, there is a twelve-month wait for a second cycle, but again things were fast-tracked because of my circumstances. And the first embryo transfer of the second harvest was successful. We discovered Hannah was pregnant within two weeks. We broke the news to our parents around the four-week mark, siblings around eight weeks, then made it public at three months.

This was almost a year after relapse—more than a year since we had walked around Cornwall Park dreaming of this moment. This was a whole new phase of life for us. That said, I am a typical guy. I am a pragmatist. And I am a doctor. I admit I did not have the passion for this particular dream that Hannah did—at the start. From my perspective, this was about me giving her the dream she wanted. But . . . things change. I knew this so well. Except this time, things changed for the better—far more than I would have anticipated. When life is suddenly created in your midst, particularly in the face of so much that has been about death and dying, you very quickly feel the significance of the moment and the miracle of creation, right in the darkest of times. I was excited. This was my dream, too. And to know it was about to come to fruition made it all the more significant.

There are so many reasons to be cautious about bringing a child into the world. Potential parents talk about their fears concerning the degradation of the environment, global conflicts, population numbers or lack of opportunities. Children born into the present world face so many more challenges than I did, or than Hannah did. And our child . . . what would our child face? We weighed this up. Neither Hannah nor I do life flippantly. We knew our child would be born into abnormal circumstances, in some respects. In others, the circumstances were perfectly ideal. Children grow up in single-parent households all the time. Most kids grow up with far less than our child would grow up with. He or she would not be any more deprived than any other human being who comes into this world. But yes, our child would grow up in a slightly different situation to the typical, clichéd home life. We weighed up these risks and we both felt, absolutely, that pursuing the dream was worth it. But this was easier to say for me than for Hannah. I would not be around on hard days or sick days or when our child needed help with his or her homework. Then again, I would not get to enjoy those times either. Whichever way I looked at it, this was more about Hannah than me. I had always considered having kids. The idea of being a dad was in the long-term vision of my life, but we no longer had that long-term vision. My view had been that children would fit around whatever it was that we were being called to do at that particular point in time—but this amount of flexibility was no longer available to us.

There was another factor to assess carefully. My bowel cancer had a complex genetic component, which meant that any child of mine potentially carried the same risk. We were aware of this from the start, even back in the idyll of Cornwall Park. We knew the risk and we knew it would necessitate five-yearly checks for our child after the age of eighteen. Was it difficult to go ahead knowing the risk? Not really. Medicine is advancing well enough that in twenty years' time, if it ever becomes an issue, we will be a lot better equipped to deal with whatever presents itself than we are now.

Some people bring children into the world without a second thought of the potential impact on them, or the risk to the child. Other children are born by accident. Some people refuse to have children at all because of the inconvenience or disruption it would cause to their way of life. Everyone is different. Every child is born into unique circumstances and for different reasons. And life is unfair, in spite of whatever care you might take to minimise the risks. That much I knew for certain. Our child would be no different. The situation was unique, certainly. Dad would not be around for much of the child's life, but the child would be born because of love, and into love. The love of an extended family would be there from the beginning, no matter what. And as the fulfilment of a dream that had never wavered, despite the challenges that had formed the backdrop to that dream, this child would carry a unique legacy into a future that I could no longer hope to have myself. As the pregnancy developed, so did this sense that part of me was going to live on. This thought was truly invigorating—and produced a determination in me to keep holding out for more. More, and more, of life.

So 2013 began with some hope; 2012 had begun with hope, too, but this was of a different calibre. I was back on chemo, notching up rounds 50, 51, 52 and up. It was a time of reflection, I remember. While the IVF program had begun, and while I had come to terms with the bad news of the previous year and found that peace I think of as being quite supernatural, I still had moments when I wished it could all have been different. I have always had a heightened sense of what it is that makes life so worth living—an acute desire to experience those things for which we live at all. And I was still experiencing these—work, travel, marriage, community, media and events, and now the prospect of family. It was what it meant to be human, after all, wanting to taste life, wanting to carve out a future, hoping to avoid suffering and pain and hardship. I had not become immune to these feelings over the years. Indeed, the opposite was the case. Despite the peace I felt and the trust I was able to draw from, I was also losing nothing of the hunger to stay alive that I had always had. I remember feeling that this home had made that longing all the more profound. Now I was getting an actual taste of what that future might have been. These decisions—home, family, career—signified a longer term future. But, realistically, it was the shorter term option I was facing. In some ways, it felt like yet another carrot to me—being dangled just far enough beyond my reach to keep me moving forward, but without the possibility of ever being fully satiated. These thoughts would never last long before I remembered how fortunate I was. I was still working, where I saw patients who had it far worse than I did. I had an amazing wife who had continued to journey by my side. And I had the promise of a different kind of life in the child of whom we had dreamt and hoped to see by the beginning of the following year.

We made the pregnancy public in July 2013. I remember making the announcement in the context of the bad news of the previous months, and how this had given us a cause to celebrate. The announcement was an invitation to rejoice with us, but also to cry with us, because there was never any forgetting the sadness that went hand in hand with any piece of joy we received. I remember a text from Hannah the day she discovered the pregnancy blood test was positive: 'I can't ring you cos I'll just cry,' it read, 'I'm pregnant!' How many times had I also written a text instead of making the call because I would have been overwhelmed by emotion? These tears were different. These were tears of great blessing and hope in the face of sorrow. So many people, from the blokes at Promise Keepers to the kids at Eastercamp, the viewers of current affairs shows or listeners to the radio, and then the many thousands of people who were following my blog, had shared so much hardship with us over the years. This was a real time for tears of gladness.

How often, though, had we been hit by the juxtaposition of devastating news right alongside the hope? Too many times to count, by my reckoning. Just two weeks after announcing Hannah's pregnancy on the blog, I was admitted to hospital with severe abdominal pain. The pain had increased following my most recent infusion of chemo, which was now at round 66. The pain was so intense I worried about another bowel obstruction, or even a perforated bowel. But over the weekend that I was admitted, the pain was brought under control and I was given yet another scan to see what was going on. The scan found that there was no obstruction, but it did find a significant amount of growth in one of the nodes behind the liver since the previous scan. It also found evidence of inflammation, suggesting maybe a bleed into one of the nodes. The results were unclear, and I would not know the true cause for a couple of days.

Two days later, I received the news I had been anticipating for years. The cancer had spread—and it was no longer responding to chemo. The pain I had experienced was malignant pain from the cancer itself. We were already in uncharted territory in terms of treatment. What to do next was a best guess scenario, but it was clear the chemo would stop and they would try radiation instead. I knew, though . . . knew inside what this meant. I was going to be robbed of the chance to see my unborn child.

Not only that, I had just been offered a general surgical registrar position, which had been my goal since med school. We were on the very cusp of more and more life, yet again. Does cancer know? Does it somehow sense that we are on the verge of life and hope, then do its worst to rob us of that chance? Of course, it cannot know, but at times it feels like it. It is one of the cruel ironies of the life of a cancer sufferer—at the moment when life is about to take a new direction, it changes the rules of the game again.

A whole team of specialists got together to decide on the next step. On their instruction I did five weeks of radiation therapy. Four weeks into this treatment, I was forced to stop work because of fatigue. They radiate such a small part of your body, but the whole of you feels hammered. I got back to work around the same time I had my first follow-up scan to see how my cancer had responded to the radiation. And the news was devastating. Again.

The cancer was rampant. It had rebounded everywhere, right through the liver. The fact that this had happened in such a short space of time signified seriously rapid growth. Riddled.

All the words you hear from people who discover they have cancer everywhere and it cannot be stopped—those words now applied to me. I know how cancer grows. I looked at my own scan and knew immediately—it was not good. If it continued to grow at that rate my liver was going to be knocked out really fast.

It was the moment we had dreaded—the moment any cancer sufferer dreads, actually. It is the moment when they tell you your life span is now measured in months. But it was October. Hannah was not due until January. I needed more than 'months'. At the rate indicated by the scan, I would not be around at Christmas, let alone January. All those years I had wondered whether this would be my last Christmas—well, this was now that time. And as for my career, about to go to the next level—one more leap towards the ultimate dream—denied. Like a customs stamp disallowing my entry into the country of my dreams right on the border.

Each of these moments along the journey has been devastating in its own way, but with each one we had learnt how to handle the initial shock, then how to comfort each other and pick ourselves up again. Then we would tell family and friends. And so on it went, every single time there was a relapse. And so, again, I rang Hannah and told her to cancel her evening plans. We knew the drill. And, of course, that night there were lots of tears, as there always had been. We both knew the ramifications, but this time there was also swearing—definitely swearing— because we knew. Three or four months out from the birth, and three or four months was all I had left.

We were gutted. Cancer was winning. I would be robbed of my chance to see our child on the very last leg of the race, and that was like a knife in the soul. That is what I posted on my blog at the time. It hurt in a way I will never forget, more than the pain of any bowel obstruction or malignant tumour. I was gasping for air. This was too surreal.

We spent days telling family, friends and work colleagues. Telling other people never gets any easier over the years. You still cry with each new person you tell, caught up in their emotion as much as your own. It is the same now when I say goodbye. It is no longer my emotion that takes over, it is theirs, but I cry with them anyway. And this was no different.

But then the tears dried up. And then I went numb. Sometimes it is the only way you can cope.

We had one course of action left: a new course of chemo-therapy was planned, consisting of the drugs 5-Fluorouracil and Oxaliplatin. What we hoped was that we might establish any kind of positive response in my liver, enough to buy me some time. The big question was whether to include Avastin in the mix. It was a big deal for us—not just the money, which we could not cover ourselves, but the very real moral objections I had to paying so much just to buy a little time. Yet suddenly, time was the most precious commodity we could buy. One or even two months could make all the difference as to whether I met my daughter or not. Any time I could spend with her was worth the world to me.

I made all of this public in a blog post on October 19, 2013. It was clear to me that I had reached what I thought of as the business end of my journey with cancer. I had accepted this end for a long time. The only difference now was the daughter I had never met but already loved.

Dear Elise,
It hurt so much because we already knew you. We had watched you grow and could see your form. We knew you were a girl and could picture you in our

home. Your home. Your room, your cot, your high chair. You were no longer just a dream. You were a person. And you had already changed the focus of my life. Of both our lives. Without you in the picture, I would have said it was time to let nature take its course. No one can prolong life forever. And my time was up.

But you were *in the picture. I could not give up. Not yet. And there was one shot left. One option open to us still. Not for a cure—that prospect was well and truly gone—but to delay the inevitable, for just long enough. All we wanted was the time to let me be around when you arrived. That made all the difference. All the other deadlines, such as my life expectancy, the growth rate of the disease, all of it was acceptable. But what I could not accept was never to see you. To not be there for your birth—that was unacceptable.*

But this one shot was unrealistic. It was expensive and way beyond our capacity. And it was not even guaranteed to work. To get this one chance, this one last shot, would take something extraordinary.

But the extraordinary happened. And it happened because of an outpouring of love . . . love like you would not believe.

CHAPTER 8
A glimpse of me

We always knew it would come to this at some stage, but perhaps not so soon. For some reason it always seemed to be a few months down the track. For whatever reason, I have managed to outlive anyone's predictions for the past five years. But now the chickens seem to have come home to roost.

I intend to keep blogging through this process as I document the journey to death, and I hope and pray that it gives Elise something to read so that she can get a glimpse of who her father was.

'Oncology 24.1', The Boredom Blog, August 4, 2014

If I paused my life right now and rewound it, like an old cassette tape, I reckon I would hear the signs of that divine thread going all the way through it. You never hear it when you just hit play, because there is too much else going on in the background—too much noise. But rewind it and listen to the sound spinning backwards at great speed . . . I think you would hear quite a different tune. And I think it would be the loudest and clearest around October 2013, when Hannah and I put our pride to one side and told the New Zealand public about the mountain before us. I am not one to equate material wealth with divine blessing. And I am not one to attach the name of God to every thing I accumulate or any property I purchase. I think blessing is often experienced in very humble ways and without any material wealth at all. And sometimes we just get what we want. Even so, it is hard to recall the events of October and not attribute them to the song I hear when I put the audiotape of my life in rewind.

I am too proud to take charity. Certainly too proud to ask for it. But in the days following my blog outlining what we were facing, we were overwhelmed by messages of support, prayers and generosity. Notwithstanding my remaining concerns about the effectiveness of Avastin, and my moral objections, it became clear to us from the response of people that we would not face the challenge of funding it alone. And on the question of whether it was worthwhile privately funding a drug that did not change the outcome, the question of how long I could survive was no longer about me as much as it was about Hannah and our unborn child. So we decided to swallow principle and seek public funding. I kept in mind how I would react if a friend was asking the same of me—it was the only way I could face asking people for financial support. We would also contribute what funds we could—savings we had managed to accrue in the previous months in anticipation of Elise's birth, superannuation I might be able to cash in under the 'severe illness' clause.

On the afternoon of Tuesday, October 22, 2013, a fundraising campaign on the New Zealand crowdfunding site Givealittle went live. A close friend set up the page for us, and that morning I wrote a blog outlining what we were doing and why we were doing it. I explained that ten rounds of Avastin would cost us $60,000 and that ten rounds might extend my life by three months. That was all I needed. Even as I wrote the blog, I realised that raising $20,000 would be a significant achievement. I had raised money before, and I knew how difficult it could be, so to raise $40,000 would be unbelievable. But to raise $60,000? That was ridiculous. I honestly believed there was not a chance the campaign would be successful. I had a whole lot of feelings going on inside as two o'clock approached and I hit 'publish' on the blog post. Humility? Certainly. Embarrassment? Maybe. Hope? I was certainly hopeful enough to give it a go. There was no other option left, so it had to be done.

But then the extraordinary happened—slowly at first, then with increasing momentum as the afternoon wore on. By three o'clock, in just the first hour of the campaign, we had raised $2000–3000. I remember thinking how nice that was—but as much as it was, it did not cover the cost of a single round. My private misgivings that it would take months to raise the required amount might actually prove to be accurate. We might raise the money, but I would be dead by the time we did. Over the next couple of hours, though, the amount kept growing. Friends, and friends of friends, were 'liking' and sharing the campaign on social media, and as word spread more people donated. I kept refreshing the campaign web page just to watch the total change by the second, like a telethon tally board. All of our friends were doing the same at home. Refresh, refresh, refresh. And by ten o'clock that night, the unthinkable had occurred. We reached our target: $60,000.

What was really extraordinary, though, was that the giving did not stop. The momentum increased. We had said up-front that any extra money raised would go towards associated costs, so the total continued to climb. Then the Givealittle server crashed. The *New Zealand Herald*, the country's national daily newspaper, got wind of the story and covered it. Not only did it cover the story, it filled the entire front page of the following day's edition with it. And the total increased by another $50,000 on the back of that exposure.

One hundred thousand dollars was raised in the first 30 hours. One hundred and forty thousand was raised in 52 hours. By the time we stopped the campaign, $170,000 had been raised, plus an additional $20,000 that was donated privately. One hundred and ninety thousand dollars! It was truly surreal. I remember thinking, 'What the heck just happened?' The generosity was unprecedented. Nuts. My friends who do not profess a faith spoke about it in terms of having their faith in humanity restored. It was a testament to the goodwill in the community, the generosity that exists in society. So much money was given by people we had never met and by people we were never likely to meet. And they were not small amounts. The biggest individual Givealittle donation was $3500. The biggest anonymous donation was $2500.

It really did reduce us to tears. Hannah and I had no words. Having been overwhelmed by the meanness of cancer and the fickle nature of suffering, we had been blown away even more by grace. Of course, the reality of the situation had not gone away. There was no forgetting that the money had been raised to buy new rounds of chemo drugs. And I had still had no idea whether my cancer would respond to the treatment. But now it was possible to try.

I did not have the words at the time to describe what happened, other than to say it was the single biggest act of generosity we had ever witnessed. Neither did I have the words to express adequately our gratitude and appreciation. The scale of what took place over those few days in late October 2013, was beyond our comprehension. This all happened less than a week from the date of my initial post following the scan. Our lives had been overturned again—this time in such an amazing way. We would be forever grateful for what happened in those extraordinary 48 hours. To family, and to friends—but also to so many members of the public we had never met and would likely never meet—we wished every blessing, as they had blessed us.

I started chemo again two weeks after the campaign, still spinning from the unexpected and overwhelming outcome. Moderating this, though, was how miserable I felt, first at the thought of going back onto a new regimen of chemotherapy, then with the side effects of the drugs themselves. Hiccups, sleeping problems, then incredible fatigue, had me struggling for seven days. In my mind, I was right back at the start of the journey. Five years on and I could still remember those first infusions and how long it would take to shake off the effect of the drugs. Here I was again—still—after all this time. I had a purpose, of course, the ultimate purpose—and this drove me on—but it did not alleviate the very real, and very disconcerting, impacts of the treatment, on both me and my work.

In mid-December 2013, I had an early scan to determine whether the disease had been stabilised by the treatment. Typically, this is done after three rounds, but my scan was done after two because we knew that if there was no sign of a positive response then continuing the treatment was a waste of time, money and quality of life. But we had some good news this time—the disease was responding, significantly so. All the lesions associated with my cancer—in the liver, the retroperito-neal lymph nodes, the lungs and the mesentery—had shrunk or remained stable. This meant one thing: I was going to see my daughter. All the love and generosity that had been poured out for this one purpose was going to bear fruit. I was as thrilled for the people who had given so much as I was for Hannah and me.

What the scan could not indicate was how long I would live, or even how long I could stay on the treatment. I was suffering terrible side effects. The fatigue was worsening, I had rampant mouth ulcers, and the toxic effects of the Oxaliplatin, a chemo drug that I had always struggled with, continued to reduce the sensitivity in my fingertips, and cause low blood pressure accompanied by vertigo whenever I stood upright.

But on the positive side, the pregnancy was going well. The nursery was set up and ready, and we were now waiting for the birth, due on January 21, 2014. I hoped it would happen between rounds of chemo, so that I could be on the very top of my game when Elise finally arrived.

Back in October, back before the campaign and just a day after realising how rampant the cancer had become, Hannah and I had driven to a beach on the west coast of the North Island. It was a blustery day, but we stayed there while we processed what impact the news would have on us, and also on our new family. One of the things we needed to talk about was the name of our daughter. This had been an ongoing discussion between us, and we had rules of engagement to ensure the name that we settled on was one we both agreed to. We both had power of veto, for example, over the other's choices. The name could not sound terrible, could not rhyme with anything unfortunate, and could not remind us of people we did not like. That left us with a very small pool from which to choose, but we had settled on three or four and Elise was one of these. When we looked up their meanings, we discovered that Elise meant 'pledged to God'. In light of the circumstances, we felt this was the most appropriate of all the names we had chosen, because this was precisely what was happening. We were pledging Elise to God. I still did not know whether I would be around for her birth, but I knew that I would not be around for much of her life, so what else could I do but give her over to God? For me, the name of my daughter was my pledge. It was also part of the hope I carried that she would be called into a bigger vision and have the opportunity to achieve things I had been unable to. And it was the hope that the God in whom I had placed my trust for so long would prove himself trustworthy for Elise. There was a real sense that the name, and her birth, had brought the entire story to its culmination.

————————

And so 2014 began—yet another year that was beginning with hope!

The birth was just a couple of weeks away but it remained to be seen how effective the new course of chemo was proving. I had a CT scan before Christmas 2013, but did not get to have a good look until the New Year. And the good news was, the response was significant—more than that, it was actually impressive. All the cancerous lesions—in my liver, my lungs, the mesentery and the retroperitoneum—had shrunk or remained stable. There was no new disease. It was about as good as we could have hoped for. There was always a chance that the chemo would have had no effect, in which case I would not have made it to the birth. There might have been a partial response, and it would have been touch and go whether I would have seen Elise. But a significant response was the best possible outcome. And more significantly, this had shown after just four weeks, which represented early response—even better!

I knew from my reading of the scan that this meant I would be around for the birth. Not only that, I would be around for a significant part of Elise's first months in the world. I would get time with my daughter.

There were other complicating factors with the drugs, which removed any certainty about how long I might have. There were questions regarding how long I could continue on Oxaliplatin, the most toxic of the drugs I was on. I knew I could not sustain ten rounds at full dose. On top of that, round five had been deferred because of a condition called neutropenia, picked up in a blood test the day before chemo was meant to happen. This explained my worse than average fatigue over recent weeks, and also meant chemo would be delayed—more well time! As ever, my life was being lived in the context of constant reminders that my body was dying. Christmas Day had been the first day in ten that I could eat without pain in my mouth from the rampant ulcers caused by the neutropenia. And I was hanging onto life because of drugs that were proving ever more toxic to my body. But . . . I was alive. And I was about to be present at the birth of my child.

And so Elise Alexandra Grace Noel came into the world, at 6.55 a.m. on January 17, 2014, weighing 3.865 kilograms (8 pounds, 8 ounces). The irony that Hannah's body was producing life while mine was surrendering it escaped me on the day, but I have reflected on it in the months since. All the way along, the themes of life and death have converged in my story, and this was no different—except that this felt like a big victory. Tempering it was the question of how long I could enjoy this new phase, but in the moment, the birth of a child signified that we had defied the odds again. Just a few months earlier, this moment was never going to be. But cancer had not won this time. Love had won.

Elise was born into a brand-new life arrangement for Hannah and me. Hannah started maternity leave in December and I was no longer working, so January was a rare month off together. It was like an extended summer holiday. And then the day itself arrived. Hannah was booked for an induction to ensure the birth fell at a time when I was well, and at six o'clock on the evening of 16 January, the procedure began. By midnight there were no signs of labour, so I came home from the hospital knowing Hannah would get in touch if contractions started. Sure enough, I got notification just after four in the morning, by which time she was well on the way. I gunned it along the motorway and got back to the hospital just five minutes before the obstetrician arrived. Labour was well advanced. I have been to plenty of births, and after observing me in action for a while the obstetrician asked if I wanted to help deliver the baby. Of course I did! I pulled on the gown and gloves, and after he had delivered the head, he let me deliver the body. Elise entered the world at five minutes to seven—a total labour of two hours and fifty-five minutes.

A lot of people talk about birth and meeting the new baby for the first time and how they did not think they could love this child more in that moment—an instant love for the baby. I did not get that moment, to be honest. To a certain extent, the birth process becomes somewhat clinical for a doctor, even this particular birth and all its associated drama. When people ask what it is like to hold that baby for the first time, I think,

'Meh! I was just holding a baby.' But once I had de-gowned and de-gloved, and was holding Elise against my skin, for me that was the moment. That was when it hit me that I was holding my daughter. Nothing, not even death, could take that moment away from me now. This was our baby, our dreams made real. I had seen her, held her, known her.

This moment lasted, and developed progressively for me over the next three, four or five weeks. As we began to care for Elise, nurture her, see her develop, that is when I began to love her more and more. I had marvelled when she was in utero—at the creation of this foetus inside Hannah's belly, and at the development of new life. I marvelled at that as much as I marvelled at the actual birth. But at the moment of connection between us, and then afterwards in the unfolding of my duties and responsibilities as a parent . . . that was when love for her became so vital for me.

And life continued, as it always had. My sixth round of Avastin was scheduled for a couple of weeks following the birth. Elise came along with us to chemo and charmed all the nurses. This was my 80th round of chemotherapy. It was not clear why I had survived for so long on chemo—but with Elise on the scene the impetus to hang around for as long as I could gathered momentum.

A week after the birth we appeared on the front page of the *New Zealand Herald* again—this time to thank and acknowledge everyone for their part in making this dream come true. I was alive because of the chemo, obviously, but I was also alive because of the public's generosity, and it was important for us to thank everyone publicly. Once again, the forum was the front page of the national daily newspaper, but we determined to limit our exposure to the media from this point on. Because the truth was, my time was limited and I wanted to spend as much of it as I could with Elise, who was the reason I was alive. It was in the context of gestating new life that I had pursued more of my own.

I watched as she became accustomed to her new world. She was immediately a good sleeper. She was not too demanding in her milk consumption. Our babymoon period of parenting was, in most ways, ideal, and I was able to see it with my own eyes and hold her in my own arms.

I will be forever grateful for her, and to those who enabled this to happen.

———————

In the weeks following Elise's birth, I was determined to not let chemo diminish my experience of being a dad. Round 80 was also the first round I endured as a father. Each round of chemo had rendered me pretty useless for several days at a time, but up until now it was something that was easy enough to deal with. I could go to bed and sleep it off, and Hannah would just feed me small amounts of easy-to-digest food over a few days. But Elise was now part of the household—and there were increased responsibilities that were far more challenging for me to uphold over those days. We were inundated with support from friends over those first weeks. We literally had not cooked a meal since Elise was born. But there were several days when I found that parenting, for me, was impossible because of the effects of the chemo. Days one to three I lost almost completely due to sleep. Hannah took on all the parenting duties then. Days four to five, I started to feel better—but even pacing with Elise would wear me out. I so wanted to be a parent, but was adding so little of value. By day six I was generally well again, and could resume my normal responsibilities.

It was like this every two weeks—normal life punctuated by ongoing chemotherapy. But . . . it had not stopped me from graduating from med school. It had not prevented me from working as a doctor for three years. And it had not stopped me from living my life—travelling, speaking, writing, being a husband. It would not stop me from being the best father I could be.

It was in this context that I remember holding Elise in my arms as she fell asleep, feeling that there was nothing to compare to this in all the experiences I had ever had. To have a child find peace in your arms . . . is there anything more magical in the world? And then she opens her eyes and stares into yours . . . And that was when it happened. That was when the whole story of my life turned and the question 'Who am I?' stopped being so important. Those eyes made me realise there was a whole new purpose to living, because of all the people in my life who had helped me be who I was, there was one person who did not yet know *me*. And that was Elise.

As Elise stared up at me, I allowed myself to imagine that she was forming memories of me, memories she could draw on in future days when her dad was no longer around. I knew it was not the case, of course, but I gave myself the freedom to romanticise for just a moment. The truth was, it was too much to admit that Elise would only ever know me through photos and stories. In some ways, this new dilemma has driven me in the last few months of my life. I pushed myself through chemo to extend my life as long as I could with this one, main objective: I wanted my daughter to know me.

To know and to be known—it is a fundamental need for all human beings. We do not grow unless we are known, and unless the bonds of love are formed between baby and parent.

We cannot thrive without relationships of love and trust. It is what every one of us desires. We know how great it feels when it happens, and how miserable life can be when it is denied us. To be noticed in a crowd. To have someone tell our story. To get a wave from someone across a crowded café. To be seen, singled out, recognised. We spend our whole lives trying to achieve it, that experience of mutuality, discovering ourselves in the knowing gaze of another.

I knew my daughter. I had been there for her birth and I was holding her in my arms as any regular father would. The overwhelming grace of the public had ensured that. But would she know me?

I have referred to the family photo up on the wall. It was taken a couple of weeks after Elise's birth and shows the three of us—Hannah, Elise and me—looking oblivious to the sadness that was about to crowd in on our home. We were not oblivious, of course, but the camera does lie sometimes. I look well. I am a good colour, have some weight, have that boyish smile about me. We look complete. The photo is bright and full of air; we have on our sparkling white shirts. It was a different time, a different place, a different health, a different mentality, but it was only six months ago. That Jared certainly looks happier than me. I always found him to be a pretty jovial character—light-hearted, extroverted, with a black sense of humour. He liked to shock people with his honesty, perhaps a bit much sometimes. You knew that when he was in the room there was always the chance of a conversation stopper. The medication has taken a lot of that away, or dulled it down at least. And the disease has taken the fat from his face and his shoulders. His hair was already damaged from the cumulative affects of years of chemo, but it still looked healthier then. He had not grown a beard and did not have dark eyes. He did not suffer the tumour sweats or the constant belching. And he was pink, not yellow.

And you can see the light of life in his eyes. Not his own life, but Elise's.

———————

I began then to imagine what 40 years with Elise would look like, and to wonder what sort of father I would have been. I have been thinking about those hypothetical 40 years right up until the present time.

Her formative years would have been very interesting. She entered a unique household, with both her mum and dad as doctors. I think she might have realised that when we started to teach her the parts of the body. I would have taught her about the arm and the leg and the head, but also the spleen and the liver. I would not have been the type of dad to rush in around her when she got a minor bump or scrape and make a big deal out of it. I would have been the type of dad who said, 'Look, it's okay, it's only a bump, you can keep doing what you're doing and you don't have to keep crying.' Life will always have its share of bumps and bruises in different forms, and that is okay. Not everything will go Elise's way. She will have bumps and scrapes like every other kid.

Even in her first few months, I liked to get down on Elise's level and play with her as much as I could. She loved books from a very early age—she would sit and listen and look at the pictures even as a baby. We had to buy books continuously because she got sick of reading the same ones so quickly. Reading is something I would have encouraged Elise to do right through life. I would want her to read whatever took her fancy—but also the stuff that takes work. I would have encouraged her to expand her mind as much as she could, with fiction and non-fiction, biographies and reference books.

If I had remained well, the time I could have spent at home would have been limited by my work. In some ways, those first few months at home were quite unreal. Medicine, for me, was more than a job, and the lifestyle it demands would have kept me away from the home for up to 90 hours a week. I would not have been the conventional dad who is home every night. In an ideal world, I would spend every minute of my day with Elise—I got very used to being able to be with her every day in her first months—but in reality, as a general surgeon, our times together would have been on the weekend. Daddy time in her early years would have been quite rare, but I think it would have been more special because of that. We would have made the most of those times and they would have given us moments to treasure, and to look forward to.

One thing I would have worked on as Elise grew up is broadening her world view. I would have tried to help her to understand that just because we grow up in a white, middle-class New Zealand, does not mean this is the only way there is to live. There are other people with different points of view, and I want her to discover why they see the world differently to her. I want her to see that most of the rest of the world lives in cultures and with lifestyles that are completely different to hers. I want her to travel, to experience those cultures first hand, to see what it is like and to get a feel for God's creation.

Elise is just one tiny piece of a big, big mosaic, one that she can go and explore and discover and enjoy. And when she understands the world on that bigger level, she will be able to chase the things she is passionate about on that bigger stage. I only knew I was passionate about the Third World when I went there. Elise may not discover the things she wants to do with the rest of her life until she has read about the world, then experienced it, for herself.

I will not be around when Elise discovers one of the more difficult aspects of life: relationships. A good father is someone who is around to help a daughter navigate those things. Relationships will be vital as she makes her way down this road. I was surrounded by wonderful relationships with incredible people as I navigated the past few years. I could not have done any of it without them. But any child has to learn for herself the same lessons that have been learnt by previous generations. It would be great to say to her now, while she is in my arms, 'Don't do this' or 'Don't do that', but the truth is, she will have to learn all of that for herself. Unfortunately. There is no other way to really know it.

But relationships will never define Elise. She will define the relationship. What I mean is that there will be relationships and friendships she has in life that are destructive. Or they will be bad influences. Or they will make her think terrible things about herself. But others will be constructive. They will be the ones that build her up and encourage her to be more than she can be, or more than she thinks she can be. They will encourage her to reach beyond herself. When it comes to romantic relationships, there is much that I would have said along the way. I would have been a very attentive dad when it came to the subject of Elise falling in love. Who she will spend the rest of her life with is one of the most important decisions she will make. I read a great quote once about romantic relationships. It went along the lines of, imagine the person that you want to be with. Now imagine that person and who they would want to be with—and ask yourself, are you that person? It makes you realise that before you go into a relationship, you should really do some work on yourself first. I wish I could be there when this happens for Elise, so that I could tell whoever she chooses that she is a person in her own right, with her own hopes and dreams.

I would say the same to Elise. A true friend is someone who stands beside them through all times, thick and thin—when things go well, and when things go bad. A true friend puts the other person first. You do not use a friend for your own advantage.

Mostly, I wish I could be there throughout Elise's life to tell her that her key relationship will be with Hannah. The circumstances in which she was born are so different that her relationship with Hannah needs to be different as well. It probably needs to be more respectful, and a bit more of a partnership. Without me around, Elise will be helping her mum get through, just as Hannah will be helping her get through.

Elise made me realise that I would like to hang around a bit longer yet. But however she comes to know me, I hope that she will also know how much I love her. Who knows? Perhaps one day she will recall an image from this time, and wonder who the bearded guy with glasses was, and why it was that he was always upstairs sitting in bed.

And then perhaps she will remember the day I was no longer here. And that may be the moment when it all clicks into place, when her dad is no longer represented by just pictures and stories, but by an actual memory of someone who held her and read stories to her, and looked into her eyes praying that one day a moment such as this would bring him to life in her memory, and give him a second chance at being her dad.

CHAPTER 9
Tunnel without a light

Getting sick is a lot like riding a train into a dark tunnel. It's dark and a bit (or maybe a lot) miserable when you first ride into it, but in the distance is a light. That light is what you are targeting; it is what represents coming out the other end—getting better.

When you are palliative, there is no light in the tunnel. You go into the tunnel, become enveloped by darkness, but don't have anywhere to go, no light so to speak. Each day is a progressive deterioration on the previous day—there is no hope that I'm going to get better. The focus is instead keeping me as comfortable as possible.

It's a bit of a major mind shift, because every other time I have been sick, there has been a light. Sometimes dim . . . but still a light.

'Palliative care 1.0', The Boredom Blog, August 30, 2014

When you are first given a terminal diagnosis, and once the initial shock has worn off, there is a period when you can suspend disbelief and live quite normally, knowing that the bad news will not come into effect until some much later date. It is like being told you need to have your tooth taken out, but the next available appointment with the dentist is some weeks away. Your tongue might accidentally hit your bad tooth from time to time, and you may even feel some pain, but by and large you have the ability to deny the reality and live as normal. Until the night before the procedure. Then there is a day of reckoning, a time when the bad news becomes actualised, the moment when you can deny it no longer.

I knew six years ago that, at some point, my terminal disease would bring an early end to my life. I also knew that, in all likelihood, in the months leading up to the actual terminus, I would confront a series of closed doors as I reached the end of the line in the different spheres of my life—personal, professional, collegial, ecclesial. With the discovery of aggressive and rampant cancer less than a year ago, I knew that those doors were beginning to swing shut. I knew the end was approaching, that the fixed-term loan of life implicit in the diagnosis all those years before was about to be called in. Even as Elise was entering this world and as we experienced all the attendant joys and celebration, I was always aware of other things coming to an end, things that I loved. Again, there was a juxtaposition of life's dramatic moments—birth and death, life and loss, hellos and goodbyes, glory and brokenness, suffering and hope. A beginning. And an end.

The first real sign that the doors were closing was in early November, while we were still buzzing from the overwhelming result of the Givealittle campaign. I began my new chemo regime as planned, in anticipation of a positive response and the chance to see the birth of Elise. There was a newfound sense, thanks to the generosity of the New Zealand and international public, that other people, both those we knew and those we had never known, were journeying with us. This sense was profound. But then I began chemo. On the day of the infusion, I felt okay. I was hoping this meant that it would not be as bad as I remembered. On the second day, I got the hiccups. For eight hours. Hiccups are okay when you have them for a minute or two, but they are a torment if you have them for a full day. You cannot sleep. Your muscles and chest become sore. And you become exhausted. They are caused because of irritation of the diaphragm, and because of nausea. I have tried every remedy, to no avail. You just have to wait them out. And it is only when they finally relent that you are able to sleep.

But then sleep is interrupted from side effects associated with Avastin. It can cause tumour pain, and this would wake me up at three in the morning. It was treated pretty well with potent pain relief, but the pain would last for days. The biggest side effect I had to deal with, though, was extreme fatigue— similar to what I am feeling now, the sense that no matter how much sleep you get you just do not feel refreshed. Each infusion took place on a Wednesday, which I anticipated would take me out until Sunday—then back to work Monday. After the first round I found it hard to get back to work by the following Wednesday. I had round two a couple of weeks later—again, out of play Thursday, Friday, Saturday, Sunday. Come Monday, there was no way I was up to going to work. Come Tuesday, same deal. Come Wednesday, I had been off work for a week and I was starting to come right. But I also realised that I was beginning to have more time off work than on, which made it very difficult to do the job. I had to get back to work. So I went through my normal morning routine. I was five minutes away from jumping in the car when the realisation hit me—I would not be going to work. I was too exhausted. Feeling absolutely rubbish. It was another moment of truth, a very bleak one. I knew that I could not keep doing this.

In the back of my mind, as a doctor, was the ongoing question of whether I was well enough to do the job properly at all. It is in the back of every doctor's mind—are you doing your very best? And I would never want to put a patient's welfare in danger because of my own ambition, in the face of my own declining health. So I just knew that this was the end. If I could not recover adequately enough even to get in the car, I could not do my job. It was the first step in a whole new phase of the sickness journey. Or, as I said in my blog at the time, it was the beginning of the end—the downhill slide to the bottom.

I loved my job from day one. After a seventeen-hour shift in an operating theatre I would still feel energised. At the time I realised it was over, I was a senior house officer. I worked on the wards but I had an informal role as a junior registrar as well. Another house officer did most of the ward work, and I got to go to clinics and assist with surgery. It was a role that did not exist on paper but was created for me, one of those situations where it pays to know the right people—and to have those people understand your situation. But I had been given a non-training surgical registrar position that was meant to start the following month. I did not know how many others had been given a position in the hospital that year, but not everyone I knew who had applied got a job. The numbers were slim. But I managed to get it, despite my sickness. It was going to be the beginning of my path towards becoming a fully trained surgeon.

The type of person who becomes a surgeon knows that it will take up a significant part of their life. I have already said that being a surgeon is a lifestyle, not a job. Some jobs support lifestyles.

This is the other way round. And you have to love the lifestyle. I knew what that meant in terms of life with a new daughter, but Hannah and I were already prepared for this. I knew it would be common for me to work from seven in the morning to ten at night—a full-time surgical trainee could expect to do 70 hours every week. So it takes a particular type of person—a really driven person. The stereotypical surgeon is someone who struggles with people skills, but I had met some lovely surgeons, people I knew were doing it because it was their passion. They wanted to be the very best they could be, and so did I.

This was my path. And just two weeks before I was about to take the first step, I knew it was not going to happen. I made the call to stop working. My sickness was infringing on the job too much. Of all the things that cancer had taken from me, up until that point it had not taken my job. When I realised that it was, finally, winning in this area too, there were more tears. For someone not given to showing emotion, this journey had featured plenty of it. I wrote an email to my colleagues that weekend, acknowledging all the people who had gone out of their way to enable me to achieve what I had achieved in the professional sphere. Again, more tears. I wept from the first word to the last. It felt like I was admitting defeat.

Beyond the job, beyond the lifestyle, beyond the calling, medicine had been a beacon. It had been something to strive for, something to achieve in, and it was something I did well. It was a big part of who I was. Despite everything, in reality I had not lost too much to cancer. Not yet. But I was losing this, and it was very hard to take.

I ended the email to my colleagues with these words:

I wanted to send this email because there have been many many people to whom I am so incredibly grateful for their contribution to either my medical care or my professional career. These people consist of surgeons who have operated on me, and those I have operated alongside; those who have treated me clinically; colleagues I have worked alongside; and referees that have helped enable me to be offered the job that ultimately I will never start. The journey over the past five years since my initial diagnosis has been difficult, but to be able to continue to study and then work in an area I am so passionate about has, I am certain, enabled me to survive longer than anyone could have predicted.

There is no doubt I am a statistical outlier, and perhaps we will never know why, but my hope is that I might continue to be one. The decision to take indefinite leave rather than resigning was with the faint hope that maybe one day I might step back into the role of the doctor, but all things being equal, I feel that I have likely treated my last patient.

We are all dealt different cards in our lives, and I want to thank you all from the bottom of my heart as you have helped me play my hand the best way I know how.

Humbly grateful,

Jared

I took indefinite leave from my job in November 2013. I suspected I would never return to the hospital in a professional capacity, but the opportunity was there if things improved. They never did. In the meantime, I continued with my rounds of chemo, then entered 2014 with my mind very much on the birth—but also with this knowledge that the doors were closing and the end was approaching. There was some fear around that for me as well. If cancer was beating me here, in my work, where would it beat me next?

I knew we were venturing into new territory, and my fear was the fear of the unknown. Tempering this was the knowledge that I would be venturing out with Hannah, and that we would at least be able to spend time with each other now that I had finished work and she was on maternity leave. The few weeks we had together in January before the birth signalled the first stage of this, and so we really made the most of that time, valuing each day so much more than we might have done in more ordinary circumstances.

But the metaphor of the tunnel began to emerge during this time, too. While normally the light at the end of the tunnel, however faint, had given me something to aim for and an exit to strive towards, this time it felt like I was just stumbling along in the dark, moving aimlessly. There was no way I was getting better, for one thing. And in all likelihood no way I would be returning to my job. There was no vision to drive towards. Perhaps not even any hope.

In truth, I have been in the tunnel ever since. That became more and more obvious as time went on, and you could say that here, at the end, I have finally reached the far wall of the tunnel where the exit is meant to be. But it was back at the start of the year when I first saw the darkness approaching.

Meanwhile, there was a semblance of normality in the Noel house. We experienced life with a baby for the first time, a phase of life we had hardly dared imagine. It was a brand-new honeymoon phase, in some ways, both of us at home experiencing for ourselves the joys and challenges of caring for a newborn.

At first it was all about finding routines and settling into them. It helped to have the model baby, something both Hannah and I were very proud of and unjustifiably took credit for! We also realised it had very little to do with us and that Elise was just pretty perfect. She would sleep in almost any environment, with any level of noise, so for that first few months she slept downstairs while Hannah and I chatted and did our regular thing around her. Then she moved into this room, into her cot, and then finally shifted to her own room. She was doing so well we decided on a road trip, which turned out to be Hannah's and my final adventure together. How fitting that we got to have at least one adventure as a family. We could not have 40 years of adventures as we had planned, but we could at least trip around the North Island. We were also camp doctors to 5000 kids at the annual Eastercamp, at which I had been a guest speaker for years. We followed this with a seven-day autumnal escape to the stunning Queenstown in the South Island.

The rest of the time was about marking moments of joy. Stable disease once again allowed me to extend the honeymoon phase. I had about five months of it. I knew I was going to get sick at some point, of course, I just had no idea when, and no idea how. Your mind puts this to one side, I think, in order to cope. You just refuse to think about it. If you worry about whether it is tomorrow, or next week, or next month, you go nuts. Even so, it never goes away, that knowledge that you are dying. It is like that hole in your tooth—always there, always making itself felt, a nuisance, really, more than anything. Until it flares up again. I think I suspended reality for days at a time, neglected to remember that I was sick. There was a sense that I should be using the time in more productive ways—writing and blogging more, perhaps. I wanted to examine some of the ideas I had flirted with in my blog and dig a little deeper into what I had discovered along my way, but I knew time was so limited that although I could be writing and producing, there was this other sense of wanting to just enjoy life for a change. To live in the now, not the future or the past. Enjoy my wife and my daughter and treasure those times.

In another sense, that sounds far more noble than what the reality actually was, because the truth is I also took the time to be lazy. What better time to be lazy than right before you die?

It was in this context that the impact of the chemotherapy upon even my most basic functioning fully hit me. The cancer had taken my profession and my calling—now it was taking the feeling from my fingers and scorching the inside of my mouth. Peeling a sticker from an apple proved far more difficult than it ever had. The numbness in the ends of my fingers meant it was an exercise in visual acuity rather than touch. Biting into the apple would make me wince, as the acid and the texture burnt against the epithelial cells of my mouth that had eroded into ulcers because of the chemo. I would clean my teeth but the white froth from the toothpaste was streaked with red from gums that could not repair themselves as quickly as the chemo destroyed them. I would make a coffee to give me a boost from the fatigue that I would feel from the night before, and taking the cap off a milk bottle was like trying to rotate a cog that would not budge. The subcutaneous tissue of my hands and feet was constantly inflamed, swollen and angry-looking.

But that is when I would sip my coffee and take a breath . . . and remember that at least I was alive to experience such things.

It was easy for me to see how quickly and to what degree chemo had impacted upon my life. I could easily make a tally of all the things that were not the same on chemo as they had been before. And I could very easily lament their loss. I realised that I was long past the prime of my life—even though it should have been ahead of me—but I could not mourn those things. If I did, I would have quickly spiralled into darkness. And so I chose not to. The tunnel was closing in, most certainly, but I chose to focus on the fact that at least I was feeling something. And at least chemo had given me a routine to hang onto.

———————

There was more media during this time. The *20/20* team returned and did a follow-up story on us, which aired in February 2014. Their coverage had begun the year before when we announced the pregnancy. They had followed the story the whole way through, and their final piece was a conclusion to the events surrounding the campaign and Elise's birth. It, too, signalled the drawing to a close of a period of life I had known for some three or four years—the period in which I had been telling my story on television and to audiences around the country. There had been a lot of media around the time of the campaign, but following our conscious decision to pull out of the limelight for the sake of Elise's privacy, that exposure had become only a trickle. All that remained of my work in this regard was the blog.

There was one final piece of print media to be published in that period, and the magazine has been by my side since the day I came home. It sits on the table on the far side of the bed—Hannah's side—but I have found myself drawn back to it in these past four weeks. On the cover, our headline reads: 'Message to my girl: Jared Noel's legacy for his daughter'. I guess it became a kind of manifesto of my final months.

And perhaps I go back to it to remind myself what remains, and what continues to be important to us right up until the end.

The magazine is *OHbaby!*, which published an article on us in April 2014. Their question, as mine had been, was how our little family would adjust to this new time, post-birth, and what values we hoped to instil in our newborn daughter. It reprints a letter I wrote to Elise, a parting note, so to speak, from a father to the daughter who would have no living memories of him. It also quotes a Bible verse, from the Old Testament book of Micah, a verse in which Hannah and I found some common ground when we shared with each other our own thoughts on values. It had been one of her favourite passages for ages, and I came to adopt it as a summary statement of the values I have had from well before I ever came across the verse. It talks about what God wants from people: for them to act justly, to love mercy and to walk humbly. They are values I have embraced and lived by since before my diagnosis. These values were the root of my calling and desire to make a difference in the world, and the reason I continued to challenge the status quo well into the days of my illness. We do not choose our values. They become apparent through our words and actions. We are what we love, and other people often see those things before we do. I hope that people have seen these values in my life. And I hope, in some ways, that Elise gets to see them, too.

Justice.

I hate to see unjust situations prevailing around the globe, and in my own life and the lives around me. When I returned from the developing world I could not reconcile how people lived in such conditions. More than that, I could not reconcile why I should live in relative wealth just because of where I was born. My hunger for justice stirred in me the desire to reach beyond myself and try to make it right—not just to make a difference, but to make it right. I never knew until I left New Zealand and saw these conditions just how lucky I was to be living here. I watched the New Zealand election coverage with Dad on the weekend and it occurred to me how much energy and time we put into complaining about the way things are. But those people who complain have no idea how good we have it compared with the rest of the world.

Mercy.

The outworking of justice. The response of love. Mercy is justice in action—actually engaging with the suffering of other people. I remember the young meth addict detoxing in the emergency department. Injustice puts her in that position. Her drug addiction was unjust. Mercy steps into that situation and demonstrates compassion.

Walking humbly.

Do these things without arrogance, or without power, or without expectation. Humility is about service, and seeing yourself in the light of other people's needs, whether that is going overseas to work in the developing world or sharing a story of how to endure a terminal illness so that other sufferers might find some encouragement.

In the letter to Elise published with the *OHbaby!* article, I wrote that I was unable to create a pithy saying or a three-word catchphrase by which she might live her life. Instead, I wanted to offer her a sense of identity, a sense of purpose and an understanding of where she came from.

That desire has kept me going through this season of closing doors. But it also reveals the questions that have been pressing on my heart during this time—the biggest of which is 'Who am I?' Now that my calling has gone, my profession is over, my responsibilities as a father reduced to an observational role, at best, who would Elise know me to be?

I know that had my life taken the direction I had intended, I would be quite a different person right now. You cannot experience the things I have over the past six years and not end up in a different place. Was that the real Jared, the one who was headed overseas and would find 'greatness' in his work for the developing world? My story might suggest so. My abiding desire to follow that dream might suggest so, too. But say I had the choice. Say I was given the choice right now not to die, but to go back and follow that other path, wiping out all that I have learnt in my journey over the past six years. What would I choose?

I do not want to die. I have said so again and again. But I have become who I am today because of the things I have suffered, and also the things in which I have been blessed. And I would not change that person. I would always want to remain the man I am today.

And if I could get well tomorrow, by some miraculous turn-around—what would I choose? Would I still head overseas, or would I do something else with the experiences I have accumulated? I am not so sure anymore. I would certainly need to regroup, figure out who I had become in light of surviving the disease. My life has been defined for so long by not surviving—would I no longer be the antihero? I would need to go back to the original vision, work out whether that still played a role in my life given everything that has happened. And maybe it would no longer be so relevant. Or maybe the vision would be all the more powerful in light of what I have learnt.

But I am sure of this: I would not change who I am today.

Several years ago, before I got sick, I attended a camp with the faith community I was involved with at the time. A guy I had never met had been invited along to take some sessions. He was someone who claimed to have a prophetic gift, which enabled him to speak directly to people with a fair amount of knowledge about their situation in life and their passions and goals. I am sceptical about such things, and I believe that whoever claims to have such insight needs to be right on the money before I will pay them any consideration. It was just before my trip to India, before Hannah and I were married, and he told me I had a passion for the Third World. I said, 'Yep.' First part right. Then he told me I would be travelling soon. Second part right. But then he told me that I was going to go on and become a person of influence and greatness. I never wrote down his words and so his precise vision has been lost over the years, but what I took away was that I was going to become someone who would achieve many things and influence thousands of people, both young and old alike.

I remember thinking how fun that sounded, but I had no idea what it meant. I have thought about that a lot over recent days. We tend to interpret these things in the context of our actual experience, and so I have interpreted what he said to be the blog and the speaking engagements and the media. I know there is great ambiguity with so-called words of knowledge and that we should listen to them with caution, but two things stayed with me: 'influence' and 'greatness'.

I really wish it had not meant cancer.

What is greatness anyway? I still feel that my life could have produced greater things. The debilitation of the disease was a blow between the legs when I first realised that those greater things had been put beyond my reach. I have always dreamt of 'greatness' in the sense of service. That has always been a key part of my dream. I did not want to be rich, but I wanted to do the best I could. It is difficult to separate my dream from ego. I never thought what I envisaged was egotistical, but this leaning towards greatness always hovered in the background.

In reality, it felt like I was on the verge of achieving something or doing something great and then it got shot down. That is how it felt. Could I have been in Africa right now? Probably, yes. I certainly felt capable, fearless, up to the task. I cannot remember ever doubting that I was ready to take on whatever came my way, and I do not remember that as arrogance, though I am sure others may have heard it that way. But then this came along, this other path. And take out any sense of a divine thread and you just have a sequence of bizarrely interconnected moments that resulted in people's lives being influenced anyway. Medicine, speaking, writing, media. Was it greatness? Was it accidental or divine? Who can know for sure?

Whatever it was, it was a life lived with purpose even in the face of my illness. Without purpose, which had been taking shape long before any self-proclaimed prophet looked into my eyes at a camp, I would have been a very different person. A person bereft of purpose just drifts through life, particularly when tragedy strikes. I could not let life just go by. I want extrinsic stimuli, people and projects to get me motivated. I can be lazy and gobble up time doing nothing. So what had my purpose become? Simply to be real and relatable in talking about my journey. To remain grounded and hopeful, to speak candidly about my disappointments and the struggles I was facing. Was this consistent with the prophetic word? Was this the path I was meant to travel the whole time?

Over the course of the past few weeks, I have often paused over the as yet unresolved contradiction between my calling and my eventual path. I have always been at peace about not knowing, or not reconciling, why I had such a strong vision when, in fact, the cellular mutations were already occurring and I would never get on that plane with Hannah and end up in Africa. But as I think about the person Elise will never know—in the sense of growing up with me and asking me things when her age and her maturity allow those questions to form—I am not so satisfied to let it lie. I am not seeking answers, but I wonder whether the contradiction, or at least my original vision, can be understood in a different way.

Here, in the darkness of the tunnel without a light, I picture a young guy who grows up with an acute sense of disparity between those who have lots and those who have very little. He sees poverty on a massive scale in the Philippines and cannot reconcile this with the wealth that he knows exists back home, or the idea that people with so much wealth still want even more of it. He is given a bizarre vision of a future in which he will influence people and achieve great things, and he is convinced it will be in that place, pursuing justice and mercy for the underprivileged and maligned people of the developing world. When he is called into medicine he feels that this is the vocation that will take him there. Put all those components together and you have a very clear adventure, together with a wife who shares that dream, to great destinations and ever-greater achievements.

And then this young guy gets cancer. And then he is told he is going to die.

But the vision is so clear, his passion so deep, his desire to make a difference in a way that is 'great' so strong, that even the devastating news of his terminal illness is relativised. Not insignificant by any means, but placed in the context of a life that he knows to be bigger and more complex than even his disease can negate. Perhaps this was his calling all along, to die in this way.

Perhaps the vision he had was preparatory, setting him up to be the most capable he could be in order to cope with the disease and achieve what he has.

I could have spent six years being sick. Who would have begrudged me that? But nothing of what has happened would have happened. I would not have prayed for the girl suffering meth withdrawal. I would not have spoken to an alcoholic about what purpose his life might now have. I would not have made friends with a guy in the States who beat me to the grave. And we would not have known our daughter. And knowing her removes the need to reconcile any contradictions in my journey.

The reality is, life is one great unresolved mystery. And we are all trying to unravel it—science, faith, the arts, philosophy . . .

But we never do unravel it.

———————

These last few months have been a bonus. And that is how I have treated them. As I ended 2013, knowing that the dark tunnel was approaching, I came into 2014 recognising that every moment was a piece of bonus time. The candle was burning and the flame was lingering on a very short wick.

We fell into a state of complacency, Hannah and I. I think we took it for granted that this was starting to work. And when cancer crept up on us again, we were caught out. Caught by surprise. But that happens when you are watching a little girl growing up in front of you. You easily get distracted. Caught up in the happiness. Caught up in life.

I never really thought that I was going to get beyond it this time. I always knew that it was catching up with me. So when I was admitted to hospital, I knew that this was the beginning of a downhill slide. You always resist, of course. It is our instinct to resist death and disease. But I knew.

The beginning of the end was in late June, after two weeks of nausea and vomiting caused not by a gastric ulcer as I had suspected, but by a partial blockage in the duodenum. At the time, I had completed fifteen rounds of Avastin. Round ten had come and gone, and because I was still responding it was recommended that I just keep going. That stopped when I went into hospital, but the truth is that I am still living now on the grace period the drug afforded me.

Several things occurred around that time that made me realise this was the moment to make a decision about my final days. I required a stent to open up the duodenal blockage, then I went home but returned to hospital with jaundice. A further CT scan showed two things: blockage of the bile ducts in the liver, which was responsible for my jaundice; and significant progression of the cancer in my liver over a very short period of time. The obstruction of the bile ducts in my liver required addressing, initially with a tube to enable the bile to drain out of my liver and through my skin, and then with a stent in the common bile duct to try to encourage the bile to drain internally. This last procedure caused me the most intense pain I have experienced in my life. After battling this for what seemed like hours, the only thing for the anaesthetist to do was administer an epidural, which also affected the nerves in my legs so that I was confined to bed. At the same time, I got an infection called cholangitis, which can come on rapidly and kill people quickly. I looked really sick at the time—although I did not feel like I was dying, others certainly wondered whether it was the end.

In some ways it was the end anyway. It was then that Hannah and I started to talk about palliative care. I knew that my quality of life was about to diminish. I had always battled for quality of life over quantity, apart from the obvious times such as the birth. The nail in the coffin was the recent CT scan, showing such rapid growth of the cancer over such a short period of time. More concerning was the oncologist's belief that the growth had started before I stopped the Avastin. This meant that going back onto chemo was probably going to achieve little. We had come down to the last-ditch therapies for treating my cancer. There is nothing to make certain you know the tunnel is closing in than to be told the best therapies around will probably do very little to halt your disease. Hannah and I processed what this meant. We knew that I was unlikely to see another Christmas, and that my time was probably going to be up sooner rather than later. The conversation about going palliative needed to happen.

This was not as hard to process as friends thought it would be. I had been living with this reality for almost six years. But at the same time, it was a brutal shock back into the reality I had been facing for so long. The past six months had seemed like a holiday, one in which Hannah and I were able to watch Elise's first adventures, together. Seeing her new life blossom was an awesome way to escape reality. But now the holiday was over. Some people approach their final days with bucket lists. I had nothing like that. I was grateful for the life I had lived, and had been given extraordinary opportunities to embrace it in all its beauty. God had blessed me enormously. And I planned to enjoy every last moment, savouring its delights and its low times. It was all part of the package.

I remember the night Hannah and I left the house to get the scan. I knew I was so sick that I would be admitted to hospital, but we were right here, in this room, preparing to leave. I took a look around, at our things, the photos, the artwork, and said, 'You realise this could be the last night that I was in this bed.'

The tunnel had closed in. Not only was there no way out, there was not even the room to turn around and head back the other way.

It was time to get down to the business of dying.

CHAPTER 10
Place of hope

Acknowledging, and then submitting, my reality to God is the only place I have found hope. Hope that energises me, hope that motivates me, and hope that what I do in this life is working towards something far greater than I could ever imagine.

It is by knowing my reality, rather than ignoring it, that the seed of hope grows . . .

And true hope has power far greater than fear . . . It even conquers death.

'Hope', The Boredom Blog, October 12, 2011

It was a Friday, the beginning of August, and Hannah and I sat with the palliative care and oncology teams, talking long and hard about when we should consider stopping our aggressive pursuit of quantity of life. Considering the impact of the final decision, the steps to achieving palliative care are relatively simple, it turns out. In my case, the biggest transition to make was from the hospital to the hospice. You do not go into hospice care with intravenous lines—they have to be subcutaneous only: into the skin. But subcutaneous lines are easily sorted. And the fevers I was suffering would be brought under control. All that remained was the decision.

We agreed that while I would still be treated for small things, we would no longer pursue treatment that would forsake quality of life. It was unrealistic to go back onto chemo, my oncologist said, because it was clear the cancer had stopped responding, and my overall health and fitness had deteriorated so rapidly over such a short period of time. So, just like that, I was palliative. I had stumbled into the final quarter. From now on, all our decisions would be based on quality rather than quantity of life. How short or long that would be was anyone's guess.

Hannah and I always knew that it would come to this at some stage—but perhaps not so soon. It always seemed like a few months down the track. But time was being called.

I was transferred from the hospital to the hospice by the middle of the month, once my ongoing biliary sepsis—the source of my fevers—had been treated successfully. The hospice is a pleasant, homely building that blends into the suburban street, not five minutes' drive from our house. Nice as the building is, palliative care is a dead end. And once you have entered the tunnel and know there is no way out, there is a period of . . . what would you call it? Purposelessness. When you are just a matter of months on from having missed out on taking the next step in your career, and from welcoming your daughter into the world, and from tripping around New Zealand visiting friends with your wife, sitting alone in a silent hospice room can make you a little despondent. I did not want to be in the tunnel. I knew I had to be, but I did not want it. I am not one to wait around. But it hit me that I was doing precisely that, just waiting to die. There was nothing I could do, and nothing I could say, to speed it up or slow it down. It was going to be what it was. Simple as that. It was not a very nice feeling.

I was in the hospice for two weeks before I came home. And it was there, in the silence, in my times alone, and waiting, that I began to reflect on hope. In the place I needed it the most, I remembered where in my journey I had discovered how hope is found not outside our suffering, but right in the midst of it.

———————

I wrote a blog back in October 2011 on the subject of hope, ironically just a few weeks before the conversation that would offer me so much hope began, one that ultimately proved fruitless. Hopeless. The question of hope in the context of suffering has occupied me for six years now, if not longer. As a person of faith, a key component of the central story of that faith concerns suffering—in fact, it concerns what the early believers said was God's suffering. At the core of my belief is an act of great suffering that leads to death, an act that represents love for all of humanity, all of creation, all of history. In the story, it is an act that claims to offer great hope, but many people, at least in my faith tradition, struggle to see the link between that story and their own. Even if they believe, when they are overcome by suffering in their own lives it is often difficult for them to see how faith can play a part in producing hope. For many, it simply does not—suffering indicates that something has gone wrong. Perhaps their faith was not strong enough. Perhaps they are being punished for having done something immoral. Perhaps God has failed them and was not trustworthy after all. As a thinker and blogger, but most significantly as someone who was told in his late twenties that he was dying, and as a doctor working with people day in, day out who are facing extreme suffering, and yes, death, the question of suffering and hope has been a recurring motif in my story. I needed to answer certain questions for myself, to understand what hope I could rely on. There is nothing like the news of a terminal diagnosis to make you confront your options for the life you have left. Will you capitulate to the disease and live out your remaining days hopeless and lifeless? Or will you find hope even in the darkness and keep moving forward? For me, it was not a matter of faith so much as self-preservation, the deep need I had to keep living and making the most of every moment, squeezing the last drop of life out of this gift I have been given.

I remember writing the blog out of frustration, not with the odds I was facing or the treatment, but with the type of hope people were selling. The sales pitch fell into one of two categories, typically. The first was the alternative medicine category. Some miracle cure had been discovered in India. It came with a conspiracy theory: people knew about the cure but the medical establishment had turned a blind eye. The second category was faith healing. People reeled out their favourite clichés: claim the healing and God will heal you; if you just have the faith, God will heal. Both approaches came from the same dilemma— people do not know how to respond to actual suffering and apparent hopelessness. Fear takes over and makes people cling to anything, even when the suffering is not their own. They opt for the impossible because the probable is too terrifying for them to face. I include in this a very particular Christian response that talks about the good that God will bring from your suffering and death. This is no more than an attempt to give spiritual meaning and a measure of value to your suffering, as if that would make it all worthwhile.

But it is not worthwhile. Suffering is not okay and it is never justified. And I have found hope in none of these places because they do not offer hope. Words spoken out of someone's fear, discomfort and uncertainty do not produce hope—at least not for me.

So now, as people say their final goodbyes to me, sometimes with a hint of this very human dilemma hovering over the room, or scribbled into well-meaning cards, I find these reflections to be more pertinent than ever. I am preparing for the final, final stage. The issue of where I find hope is more profound now than ever before. A day is coming when I will no longer have the capacity to think about hope or the meaning I have discovered in life. By the time that day dawns, I intend to be hope-filled, at peace with reality and steadfast in holding onto what I have learnt. I want a hope that is reliable, and by that I mean a hope born of suffering itself and not of fear.

———————

I was never on a quest to find the meaning of suffering. Nothing so noble. My own search for answers to my questions emerged organically from my situation and from witnessing so much suffering in my daily duties at the hospital. A doctor cannot ignore the actuality of suffering, but not all doctors question why or how, in a spiritual or metaphysical sense. But it is very difficult to believe in a loving God and not raise some questions when you experience suffering yourself, if only in the lives of the people around you. And the pursuit of the meaning of suffering is ancient. Humanity has always had trouble with the interface between belief and suffering. The story of Job, one of the most ancient biblical texts, is a clear example of how long we have tried to come to terms with suffering in general, and the bigger questions regarding why we suffer.

My trajectory as a blogger began by presenting the suffering I was experiencing as a cancer patient on chemo. In the early days, the whys and the wherefores did not occupy me as they did later. That came after the first relapse, when I knew my time was short. The latent questions that were probably there all along now had bite. Around that time, I wrote asking whether my diagnosis was fair, but set this question against the cases of injustice I saw happening in the world. I did not think I could really ask whether it was fair when in some instances millions of people had been wiped out at a time. Even then I knew it was a matter of perspective. I suggested that instead of wallowing in our own difficult circumstances, we should seek to be the answer to the prayers of our neighbours and friends, even strangers. I did not say it at the time, but I was already avoiding asking the question why. I found no peace in asking that question, even then. I found peace in considering how I could continue to help people in their suffering, which needed me just to accept that suffering was a part of life.

Part of this was a concern for people of faith who were besieged by doubt and anxiety over the discord between their expectations of faith and the reality that things actually do go wrong. I wanted them to know that life still goes on despite things going bad. Life will always have ups and downs, but that does not mean there is something wrong with you or something wrong with God, or something wrong with your capacity to believe. Faith is about a journey, it is not a mechanism for ensuring everything always goes according to plan. And by definition, faith makes room for doubt. If doubt does not exist then everything is self-evident and there is no need for faith. And part of what causes doubt in the human psyche is suffering.

Approaching Christmas that same year, I formulated the approach I would take throughout my journey. I realised that part of the human endeavour is the need to understand, and that so many areas of life are particularly well suited to having the why question posed of them, particularly in science. Why are plants green? Why do the stars move in the night sky with seasonal variation and repetition? Just two examples. But the why question does not apply in other areas. Just because a why question helped us discover a heliocentric universe does not mean it will help us understand why I have cancer.

I was also becoming more aware of just how broken humanity was. I seemed to see this more after periods off work because of chemo. I would return to work and recognise more potently the depths of brokenness that people have to endure. In this, I realised that some of the questions people ask about suffering are not necessarily to get an answer to the question, but to help them cope. Sometimes it is reality itself that threatens to overwhelm us. Even faith is used as a tool in this regard, concocting fanciful ideas to help us avoid the realities of this life's precarious nature.

I was experiencing the ramifications of this first hand, in the blasé comments people made to help me not lose hope. People would leap to the defence of God, not to say outright that there was a reason I was suffering, but because they were unable to accept that God was allowing the suffering to happen in the first place. They could not bear to think about the questions that scenario raised. They wanted to suggest there was some higher purpose or deeper meaning to my illness, and that I would feel God's peace and grace because of it. But I did not want to hear this. It was almost a beatification of suffering, glossing over how hard it actually is and giving it a sickly-sweet spiritualised coating, like medicine hidden in sugar.

I attended a symposium on faith and cancer during this time, and realised how the beatification of suffering was a centuries-old problem in my own faith tradition. It was often peddled by people who had not suffered or who had suffered just a little, and therefore had some academic interest but had not really wrestled with the issues themselves from the context of a life-and-death struggle. Even the passion of Christ and the tradition of the Stages of the Cross came from this sense, that it was the suffering of Christ itself that had value, and that therefore all suffering had meaning. If you suffer, you share in his sufferings, and that is somehow redemptive. It gives value and meaning and purpose to suffering. But this value is a fantasy.

What is suffering anyway? And how much suffering is enough to give it this value? Not everybody's suffering is the same. One person's suffering might be another person's misery. One person's misery might be someone else's irritation. While I have suffered during this experience, I do not believe I have truly suffered. I read about the suffering of some people in situations of persecution and torture, and I know that their experience is worse than mine. And many of them still get through it, which produces another pithy saying that has been given to me over and over: I will not be given anything that I cannot handle. This is a nice idea, but what about all the stories from around the world of people who do not get through their suffering? What about the people who actually die at the hands of suffering? We hear about the people who do overcome and their stories get told in churches in connection with these pithy sayings, but for every one of those stories there are a lot more people who are given precisely more than they can handle.

This time at home has given me opportunities to follow world affairs on television. The world is in a miserable state right now. Often throughout history there has been one major conflict going on somewhere in the world. Right now, there are multiple sites of conflict and war and suffering, atrocities occurring on a whole different level, often in the name of religion. They are some of the worst atrocities I can remember, and so many people caught up in these conflicts die. When you come across a village and there is a mass grave of 100 or more people, it is safe to say those people did not overcome their suffering. Many of them have suffered prolonged deaths at the hands of torturers.

I have come to realise that we cannot always say we will overcome the suffering we encounter. We need an understanding of suffering that accounts for the many, many people, millions of people in the current world, who will not overcome. The beatification of suffering and our pithy sayings and the notions of faith relying more on fear-based fairy stories do not take those people into account. The reality. The beatification of suffering implies that they will overcome, but worse, it suggests that such suffering is justified. And suffering that is considered justified is usually perpetuated by other people, often by those who believe they are doing God's work.

My faith has always been pragmatic. I have always looked at the reality of what is going on versus what is being preached, or taught, or peddled. If the ideology does not match the reality, something is wrong. And I have become intolerant of pithy sayings over the past six years. Even statements said in good faith and with kind hands can be damaging. They are unhelpful. And they do not generate hope. When you are lying in your bed two weeks out from death, you need more than the sanitised version of life people are prone to give you in such circumstances. You need real hope.

When I look at humanity's attempts throughout history to give a plausible answer to the question 'Why do we suffer?', matched against the answers they have come up with, I have to conclude that the question itself must be wrong. The complex frameworks that theologians and philosophers have constructed to answer the question never quite work. Even if they go some way to addressing the dilemma, none of their models go all the way. As someone who is dying, I do not need a model that goes some of the way. Some of the way is still too far away for me.

Perhaps these frameworks do not answer the question because the question is wrong from the very beginning. And perhaps the question is wrong because what the question is seeking to achieve is wrong. And what the question is seeking to do is work out the meaning of suffering. We are meaning-seeking animals, and we are consumed by the quest to find truth and meaning in all things, even suffering. This is an evolutionary reality. A primate in Africa that hears the grass rustling quickly learns what the meaning of it is—there is a tiger about to attack. That meaning only arises as a result of experience. The next time you hear the grass rustle you run. You do not need to see the tiger because you have already learnt what the noise of the grass moving means. We do this in our lives all the time. It is called psychological bias. We have many biases that allow us to draw meaning from things without having to go through all the steps to get to it. But the problem is, these biases also shortcut our way to actually acknowledging whether it is relevant information we are drawing from a new and changing world. Are we drawing conclusions and making assumptions about things without all the evidence? Have we imposed categories on things when they are not necessarily correct?

One of these false assumptions is that it is possible to find the meaning behind our suffering. The woman who says to me that God knows all things and makes all things good and will bring good things out of my suffering and that this should give me peace, has made a massive leap from a psychological bias to the meaning of my suffering. And she has done this because of fear of what my suffering actually indicates. When people see suffering, it is like the primate in the jungle, jumping to conclusions about its meaning and then running from it. They jump to conclusions about suffering itself, and about God, and about humanity, even about me and my family, my disease, the myriad of complex factors that have played a part in putting me in this room, at this time, on the verge of dying. I know from looking at the historic attempts of humanity to ask these metaphysical questions that they have taken a shortcut in the process. Even Job's friends came to him with their creative and compassionate theories for why he had suffered, each one intelligent and poetic and deeply considered—and each one of them wrong.

There came a time in my first year of chemo, perhaps around the time of my first relapse, when I knew that we needed to go back to the beginning and rethink the question. Examine the process from its origins. Apply checks and balances to the shortcuts we are making in order to come to conclusions that assuage our fears but are useless in the reality of the situation in which people like me and the patients I work with find ourselves. So now when we hear grass rustling, is it truly because there is a tiger there? Not necessarily. It might be the wind or another, less dangerous animal. Or it might be that the grass has developed the ability to move by itself.

Why do we suffer? Maybe it is an irrelevant question. Maybe the question is flawed. Why is God allowing me to die? Maybe that is an irrelevant question, too. What is the meaning of my cancer? I can guarantee that this question is not only completely irrelevant, it is also potentially damaging. To find any kind of hope in my situation, I have needed to approach this dilemma from the wholly other side.

———————

What I have come to realise is that suffering is meaningless. That is why we cannot find answers to the questions we throw at it. We struggle to find the meaning in the things we suffer because there is none there to be found. My cancer and death at the age of 32 are meaningless. They have no inherent value. I did not get sick to serve some greater purpose or because I had done something wrong. It was not to teach me a lesson. I could spend every waking moment between now and losing cognition and I still would not find the answer to the question why, because there is no answer.

But I can create meaning in the context of suffering. The meaninglessness of suffering does not have to be the final word. It is an opportunity. And that is the choice I face: succumb to the meaninglessness of this world's brokenness, or search for value in spite of it. Whether that suffering is linked to financial hardship or ill health, it is the same thing. There is no point wasting any time trying to understand their value. But to come to terms with the doors they open for even more value and meaning in your life . . . that is a different story.

I was always leaning this way in my understanding, I realise now. The typical questions just never worked. I have never encountered anyone who could give me a satisfactory answer to the question of what purpose our suffering serves. But it was not until I sat in that symposium that I could formulate the dilemma so succinctly. It made so much sense in the context of my story and the wrestles I'd had, the disappointments, the challenges and hurdles. Quite apart from the issue of my actual sickness, I had bigger unresolved issues to contend with—the loss of vision and calling, which I was sure was from God. If I had wanted to, I could have spent every moment of the past few years trying to get my head around that one, but there was no point. There was no reason why my calling had been disrupted by cancer, no meaning or explanation behind the divergent path my life needed to take. That is what suffering is. It is the imposition of meaninglessness on a life that otherwise has order and balance, goals, structures, dreams and passions, and value. It is destructive on account of the very meaninglessness inherent within it. And that is actually the greatest dilemma that confronts us. We have this meaninglessness as part of our reality, and must contend with its effects daily. Whether watching the rampant advance of the Islamic State on the evening news or dealing with the rampant growth of cancerous tumours in my abdomen, the nature of the problem is the same. Meaninglessness is part of our world.

The part of my story that still makes me smile, even now, is that I was able to experience meaning and purpose despite this, and despite what might have been overwhelming disruption to my idea of what my life was going to be. And that this happened by accident is an element of my experience that I particularly treasure.

Not everyone will sit so comfortably with the idea that suffering is meaningless. For me, it is the only way to approach the question of suffering in a way that makes complete sense.

Others will continue to struggle with the issue, and that is okay, too. They will point to the fact that I have been able to achieve things that I never thought possible, precisely because of the sickness I have been through. And that is certainly true. But I would say that wherever someone points to suffering as having created significance and meaning, I would argue that love could do the same and more. And in most situations it is probably love that has created the meaning, not the experience of suffering. And this is why admitting to myself that suffering has no meaning has made such a difference. Suffering is a vacuum, a nothing, which means it leaves room for us to create within that space. The creative response that takes up most of that space is love—going beyond yourself for the sake of others. That happened for me accidentally, as the blog generated a following and as doors began to open for me to stand before audiences and television cameras. But the impulse in me was always to reach beyond myself and make a difference in people's lives. That hunger never abated, even after being handed a terminal diagnosis. In fact, I just became more determined to make my life about other people.

In all of this, though, I have still needed to mourn. I have still needed to grieve the life and opportunities I have lost, particularly where Hannah has been concerned, and now Elise. But being able to acknowledge that suffering has no meaning has given me the freedom to grieve for those losses at the same time as continuing to find meaning in acts of love. And I have experienced more love from others than I have been able to generate for them. I have still cried. I have still felt emotion. But love has allowed me to turn my losses into something creative, something significant. A consequence of this is peace. Total peace. I will die knowing that I found meaning in the context of my dying. Despite it, in fact.

Do I feel fear? No. Fear accompanies the question why. When you no longer have that question, and experience love in its place, how can you fear?

Do I feel regret? Yes, about the things I will not be able to do with my life. But the life that I have lived already . . . I feel no regret about that. Were I given the opportunity to live another 30 or 40 years, the things that I would hope to achieve in that time, they are the things I regret.

Do I feel happy about my life? Yes, totally.

Do I feel loss? Yes, loss of the opportunities that my future will not hold, with Hannah and Elise. Loss of my calling. I will carry that loss with me into the final, final days.

———————

I have not come to this place of peace without a wrestle. At times, that wrestle has been painful. Confusing. Gut-wrenching, even. My heart was sold on the vision I had. So when I was first diagnosed, it felt like another step in the journey. It was a very big step, but a step nevertheless. But as time went on and my prognosis worsened, issues were raised that had less obvious answers. I had to really wrestle with these. It was difficult to reconcile the two things: my calling to go overseas and my terminal disease. They just did not fit. They are still unresolved. Right now, this close to death, I still have not resolved that discord. Because it cannot be resolved. That would assign meaning where none can be assigned. I just have to sit with the tension of the meaninglessness of one reality destroying the other.

What I have been given in all of this is hope. Over the course of the journey, I have experienced the types of hope that anyone in my predicament has: the hope of treatment, the hope of a cure, the hope that I would be around to see my daughter, the hope that I would get to enjoy just one more day of work. But these smaller hopes were nested inside a much bigger hope—the hope that I would be of use to other people, that the broken story I was telling them would somehow strike a chord and would make a difference, and that this difference might even have a rolling effect through the community, and the nation, and the world. This hope came to replace the more personal, selfish hope, to a large degree. I found value not in finding a cure and pursuing my own dreams, but in being rewarded with opportunities to change people's lives, in spite of my vulnerability.

I still have those personal hopes. They are no longer about a cure, because I accept my death. No, my hope is now focused more on the faith community that comes to gather around my bed, that community of friends who have travelled with me along the way. My hope is actually that I have sown a seed, and that they realise that their potential to make a difference in the world is only limited by their own understanding of the world. Things are not always going to happen in line with what they want or expect, but I hope that my story has shown them that even so, wonderful things can happen. There is always a bigger picture we cannot see. The amazing thing is that even with our limited vision, we get to play such a big part in making it happen.

I hope, too, that they spend the rest of their lives seeking to build the community and helping people to understand faith in this light—that they have within their reach the opportunities I had, regardless of circumstance. I hope they avoid getting caught up in midlife crises and materialism. I believe they will go and spend their lives making a real impact, and if not the impact measurable by typical means, certainly the sort of impact an antihero makes.

It is impossible to find meaning in the context of suffering without a community of people around you—friends, family, colleagues—people with whom you get to share experiences of love, of really reaching out beyond yourself and making a difference in their lives. And the same is true in reverse. It is impossible to keep the fires of love burning if you are not receiving it from others. To find hope in the midst of sickness and dying requires people who will journey with you. These people have journeyed with Hannah and me. They have walked so closely beside us that they have known when things are going bad and when things are going well. The value of their presence has been impossible to measure. My journey has given them pause, to think and wrestle with what life is all about, what faith is in the context of suffering, and the central place of love in the search for hope. They have wrestled with these things as much as I have. And they have not done it from a distance. They have been right there by our sides.

There is a cost to human suffering. In my case, that cost was measured in rounds of chemo, all 89 of them. That cost is fairly brutal. But love is experienced when there are people close enough to you to see what 89 rounds of chemo actually look like. And that is where you find meaning. In the love that can generate hope, no matter the circumstances and no matter how close you are to your final, final moments.

CHAPTER 11
Business of dying

———

But now the holiday is over, and I have to get back to the business of dying. I plan to do that the best way possible, as not everyone has the privilege of anticipating their own end. So often people's end times are full of regrets and catching up with bucket lists. I don't have either of those. I am grateful for the life I have lived. I have been given extraordinary opportunities to embrace it in all its beauty. God has blessed me enormously. I plan to enjoy every last moment, savour its delight and its low times. It's all part of the package.

'Oncology 24.0', The Boredom Blog, July 26, 2014

Dying follows no formula. We all die in different ways, and the person who dies in the way I have, in a drawn-out fashion, waiting for the end, will discover that changes happen daily. Your body reacts in ways no one can anticipate, and your mood follows. If spirituality is a component of your final days, that, too, is contingent on your physical state and your mental capacity, how much fatigue you feel, your patience, your level of anxiety, the amount of spare time you have between sessions of goodbyes with friends, your nausea and your symptoms of acute or general pain. There is not one way to die. And there is no manual for how to do it well. There is only the experience and what you bring to it. Fear or trust? Resistance or submission? Suffering or hope? Love or loneliness? Those things need to be in place well before the end. They are the things you should fashion and nurture and protect in life, not in death.

I have handled the business of dying pretty well, I would say. I have seen the people I have needed to see. I have always said I wanted dying to be a faith-building exercise, and I hope I have achieved that. I think I have been as transparent as I could be. I do not know how close God is, but I presume he is close. I am not feeling him, but I believe he is here.

At this moment, it comes down to handling the now and coping with the fatigue. Just trying to push through to what-ever is next. There comes a point when you just move on to the next phase. That is what follows for me. Certain things will happen that are typical for all terminal patients, peculiar little psychological and physical responses to the breaking-down of the body's mechanisms. Hand gestures. Anxiety attacks. Incoherence. Babble. Then sleep.

But in all other respects this final stage of the journey will be mine, and mine alone.

I came home on a Wednesday, unable to walk because of the paralysis caused by the intrathecal block in my back, and because of the loss of strength in my legs due to lack of use. From the start, I felt most impairment in my cognition. I had no fears about the next few weeks, and in fact remember feeling somewhat invigorated by being home and facing the challenges of this final stage. I was always aware that this could change within a day. I saw a photo of myself a couple of days after coming home. I had not realised how much weight I had lost or how different my thin, hollow face looked with a beard.

The second night home was when I fell out of bed. I have talked about moments of tears marking the most difficult periods of my story. This was another. I was never in doubt about the challenges of this final period, but this incident reminded me that despite my experience as a doctor, there would be a few challenges I could not anticipate.

The first weekend came and went without much change. We had wine and cheese with our friends on the Sunday night. I guess I felt a little wearier each day, but it was a vague feeling. I just remember that I did not seem to have as much energy as I had the day before. But we got to use the hoist on the weekend and so I had some time in the recliner rocker, and this meant I got to spend time out there in the activity of the house.

A couple of days after the weekend, though, I was feeling quite out of sorts. It was very hard to wake up. I had a wash and the exhaustion of that overwhelmed me. I had a rush of nausea and could not recover my strength. Emotionally, I was tracking okay. The exhaustion does have an impact on how emotional you feel, though. I recovered when I could by taking extended afternoon sleeps.

The following day was the first time I realised that the way I was feeling was perhaps not something I would recover from but the new normal. This was a little disconcerting. The feeling was hard to describe—just out of sorts from the moment of waking up. In the early stages, you are weighing up on a daily basis whether what you are experiencing is a temporary feeling or a result of the progressive deterioration that comes with the disease. It was impossible to predict how this would go. And there was nothing I could do to improve how I felt.

A full week after coming home, I was given some hope. Not long-term hope, of course, but some important short-term hope. I remembered that over previous days the doctor had changed a lot of my medication. It was possible that I was feeling so bad because of withdrawal. One drug had been stopped and two others reduced, so this was a real possibility. But hopeful though I was, I was also having moments of feeling very miserable. There were times when my head would just drop into my hands for ten or so minutes and I would feel awful. In such moments, I would just have to push through. But I remember thinking, just one week home and it was wearing thin already.

There were moments, too, when I could see how death would come as a relief. I had no control over that, though. Such moments would pass and I would not feel so despondent for long, but they marked my lowest points.

By the weekend, which was now my second week home, there had been no discernible improvement. In fact, things were getting worse. It was so hard to wake up. So, so hard. I still blamed the sedative effects of the medication. Or perhaps I should say that I hoped it was this. Either way, it occurred to me that we needed to roll them back even more.

The following day was Father's Day, and while I actually felt some improvement, I was fighting intense abdominal pain that we could not source. Nurses were brought in to help and we finally got on top of it, although we never did work it out. It could have been the sushi I'd had for lunch.

Over the course of the next few days, little changed. There was no improvement and the effort to wake up was getting tougher. By the Thursday of that week, a full two weeks after coming home, we decided on a bigger adjustment in medication. For one thing, the amount of drugs going into my intrathecal block would be reduced, allowing me to move about the house. And there would be an adjustment to how my methadone was administered, which hopefully would reduce my fatigue.

In the midst of this, though, I remember a tough night with Hannah. I was beginning to experience bouts of melancholy, and this would manifest in tears—when thinking about the future, mainly, and what I would miss out on by dying so young. I remember praying about how hard it was to go through what I had to. The pain. The lack of mobility. My state of mind. I was hesitant to pray for the end to come more quickly, but I wanted it to be easier and I knew it was not going to get easier. It cannot get easier. I am dying. And the prospect of that brought me to tears.

And things did get harder. Rapidly. The weekend was terrible. The Saturday was a miserable day, and for no apparent reason. The pain and nausea were very difficult to handle. Sunday was better, but I was exhausted from the challenges of the day before.

By the Monday, though, the improvements we had hoped for finally started to show. I was moving around, even if with great difficulty. Nevertheless, I had been able to get downstairs and wheel myself around. We'd had a weekend of people, too—a visit from Hannah's brother, my family over on the Sunday. I remember a conversation with Hannah over those two days, flagging that I thought this was the beginning of the downhill slide. I was in no doubt by then that what I was feeling was the gradual deterioration leading to death. I could no longer blame the medication.

And so why I felt better just one day later, I did not know. I was malnourished and my liver function was not what it should be. I was jaundiced and had experienced drainage problems with the tube in my side, but I had more energy. Perhaps we had finally landed on the right balance of medications.

I was now three weeks home. A Wednesday. September 17. The day before was my big farewell to our closest friends. I was downstairs, where I spent much of the day in the recliner feeling better than I had felt in a long, long time. But then again, just a day later, I was hammered. I woke about five in the morning, feeling ill and coughing. The rest of the day the same feeling came over me, that feeling of being non-specifically unwell. It was impossible to describe. The hospice nurse said it was usual to experience this the day after a good day, because you try to achieve so much while you are well but you always pay for it with a relapse the next day.

By the weekend, this feeling was worse. Each day was now a struggle. There were some better moments, but overall the decline was clearly mapped, so much so that the days began to blur. Frustration was what I felt the most. When you live your life being able to refresh yourself by sleeping, then here when you need it the most, the sleep just does not refresh you at all, the struggle is relentless. I was sleeping twelve hours each night and waking up as tired as when I went to bed. As a result, my mood suffered. I had experienced some very low moments, when I felt defeated. It was depressing—not in the clinical sense, but in the sense of depressed functioning, depressed thinking. The New Zealand elections were on the weekend. I peak in the evenings, typically, so I looked forward to the election results that night. Mum and Dad were here too, so we watched television together.

Sunday was even tougher than the Saturday. I was incredibly fatigued. More so than the day before. You cannot appreciate anything when you are as worn out as I was. Company makes a difference, though, even if nothing is being said. I like it when Hannah takes her downtime in here. My GP has told me I need to think of dying as an endurance race. I have to break it up into parts. How can I get through the day? How can I get through this hour? Don't think about what is ahead. Every day is a new day. Forget tomorrow. There is a Bible verse in which Jesus says something very similar. So that is what I have done. It is the only way I know to cope. I just start a day, wait to see how I feel, learn from previous days what works and what does not work, what makes me feel better and what makes me feel worse.

Now, here we are today. How do I feel today? The worst I have felt so far. Massive, massive fatigue. On a whole different scale. Brain fog, for one thing. Each day has its ups and downs. Today I think I have managed things okay, but the fatigue is increasing and will continue to do so. I have no doubt now that this is all the result of slow organ-system failure. Just as the liver begins to fail, so the organs around it begin to fail as well. Neurotoxicity results and the brain begins to not function as well as it should, simply because what needs to be cleared from the system is not being flushed away.

No one likes putting numbers on these things. No one will say when the end is likely to come, but I am saying one to two weeks. That is the barrel. That is what I am staring down.

———

At some time or other we all face our mortality. Sometimes we are confronted by it out of time, out of sequence, almost anachronistically, and we get a second chance at life. This is the 'It wasn't my time' scenario, in which people claim to have stared death in the face yet survived. Often when that happens, we see extraordinary things come from those lives, which are suddenly played out with increased intensity. There is a reason for this. Mortality heightens the senses, deepens your hunger, animates the spirit, sharpens your knowledge and your sense of what might be. It paints dreams in vivid colour, gives ballast to your determination, adds contours and texture to your desires. It takes your goals, which once seemed so far off, and brings them very close, so close you can taste and feel them. Alongside this, other feelings come into play, feelings that probably conflict with the heightened senses and animated expectations. Mortality as experienced by the terminal patient brings with it a whole host of challenges. Uncertainty plays a big role, by virtue of the fact that you simply do not know. You do not know when death will occur. You do not know whether the things you are feeling are associated with dying or with continuing and diminishing life. You do not know how difficult the end will be.

The loneliness of dying can bring its own challenges. It is an isolating process because no one else shares your experience of the tunnel in quite the same way. Most of the people around you still have no idea what it is like to be in that place with no light to guide their way. No one feels fatigue the same way, or lives with the knowledge that what they are investing in life right here, right now, is largely redundant. Everything you are contributing to life in this moment is about to fade away.

I have not been lonely in my isolation. A steady stream of visitors has brought its own demands, but they are counterbalanced by my need for people. In these times, I have often thought back over my period of clinical depression. That was when I knew real loneliness. I could not imagine going through what I am now if I were as lonely as I was then.

Nevertheless, you die alone, which means you take the final steps alone. People can walk beside you only so far. At the end of this journey is a turnstile that only one of us walks through at a time. You have to search your own soul as you near the end. No one can do this for you, either. Search your own understanding as to why you believe what it is that you believe—about your life, your journey, your relationships, about what comes after, about what you have left behind. And when your thinking takes you deeper inside yourself, make sure there are people on hand when it results in tears and sorrow. My journey would have been very different if my faith community and family and friends had not been around me. It would have been a much tougher path to tread—practically, emotionally, spiritually, relationally.

Dying has its own frame of mind, its own moods and its own humour. How can you laugh like you did when you feel so exhausted you spend an entire day trying to wake up? You cannot. And no matter how funny you are at the times when you are well, dying will test the capacity of your spirit to find relief from the heaviness. And despite the trust you might place in a bigger picture, or God, or the universe, and regardless of whether your faith remains steady to the end, you will experience periods of grief and loss, unresolved aspects of your life, moments when you want the living to end and the dying to come. My lowest time was right in the middle of this last four weeks. I was so low, so fatigued, that the thought of dying over that weekend gave me such relief. I found myself wondering why my body would not just let go. Who was it that I was holding on for? Was there something else left to tick off?

In this time, I have experienced deep sorrow. I think sorrow sits side by side with faith, or trust, or submission, or even peace. I think mortality affirms what is a fundamental truth of living. We can sorrow even as we discover hope. Our humanity is capable of great complexity when it comes to hope and loss, and I have lived with the tension of peace and sorrow for many years now. Grief is important for the person facing death. It is a vital part of the process of dying, and I have certainly gone through my moments of grief. Hannah and I cry often. The tears are mostly mine, I guess. Hannah will have a different journey that continues on without me. This experience will be a stepping stone. Her grief is no less than mine, but for me this is the last stone before I reach the other side of the river.

All the same, the sorrow does not press in on me like it might. There is nothing claustrophobic about the tunnel, no sense that death is approaching like a dark angel. There is no anxiety. At least not yet. There is no panic. It is just grief, accompanied by peace. Indeed, it is a peace that gives me the room to grieve and to sorrow for the life I will never experience, but also for a life that has been so good it deserves to be mourned, even before the end.

———————

I have accepted death and I am at peace in the face of my own mortality, but that does not mean I have accepted the way it ends. And it does not mean I would not keep striving to make this time easier, for me or for anyone else. There are things about dying that are out of our control or influence, other things we can change. Even now there are elements of this final step that I am resisting, other things I am holding out for. Death does not come as it does in *Harry Potter*, as a curtain we merely step through. It is a wrestle. A conversation. A negotiation.

I have a friend in the United States, a man who contacted me through the blog because he was going through a similar journey. We have been in touch for six months or so, and he went palliative two months before I did. I sent him a text around the time I was in the hospice. His sister replied and said he could not respond because he was on so much pain medication he was incapable of responding. You can get to the point where you are so drugged up you cannot eat or drink. And eventually that is what kills you. It has challenged me, seeing him go this way. Is that a humane way to die or not? Is there another way? I got a message three days later to say that he had died. My text to him had said, 'I'll race you to the finish line.' It seems I lost.

Even now, so close to the end, I find that as I reflect on mortality and letting go, there is life right there, standing in the way. I think perhaps this is the way it should be. Life is too precious to let go too easily or too soon. Even at these times of what I would call despair, when I have really wrestled with the issues of how to die well, and tried to fathom who it is that I am holding on so tightly for, I have always seen that there is still life that I want to live and things that I want to do. Whether it is something as significant as spending more time with Hannah, or as frivolous as hanging on for the next Apple product or *The Hobbit* movie—it generates the same fight within me.

But at the same time, it is a hard, hard slog.

I have witnessed enough end-of-life experiences to know how it goes. Strangely, though, I have not recalled those memories to help me confront my own. The first experience I had, long before any clinical experience, was the death of my grandad. I remember it clearly—it was a sight to behold. It did not bother me but I will never forget it. Since then, I have had several patients die in front of me, and it is always a memorable moment.

And despite my faith, I have not given much time to thinking about what comes next. Not even now. I think enough people have tried throughout history to contemplate what comes after, but the results have never been convincing. I will just experience it as everyone does—in due course.

But let me be clear about what I believe. We all have some belief about what comes next, even if that is nothing at all. Some people may hope there is something else without actually having any idea what it will be. I am very close now to that point of knowing. 'One step closer', so the U2 song goes. I am looking forward to the next life. I have that up my sleeve. I know there is a next life, but I have done enough reading of the Bible's prophetic texts to know that nobody really knows what it is like. People have defined subgroups within faith movements based on what they think might happen, but what it boils down to is we do not know. I am just happy to let it happen. But I know I get to rejoin my creator. I have no idea what that will look like, but that much certainty I do have.

Mortality. The great enemy. Finality. Perhaps the beginning of something else. But certainly the end of this thing.

It separates life from death. Stands there like a great barrier. Even if there is something that comes after, it only occurs on the other side of an experience that is dreadfully final. If death is hell, then we get to walk to the very gates when we die. Sometimes we walk hand in hand with others who dare to approach the gates on our behalf, like Dante's narrator being led through the inferno until he finally gets a glimpse of paradise. The idea of hell fills me with despondency. My hope most certainly lies in the other place.

From the beginning, from Diagnosis Day, I have had a heightened appreciation for life, and because of this, of death, too. It gave me a sensitivity to the spirit of life itself, its beauty, its opportunities, its complexities, its rewards. I am more aware of those things now than I ever was before, but I am sensitive to something else, too, and this is the insight that only mortality can give a person. I believe this is why so many who return from near-death experiences—not just the experiences that get trumpeted as spiritual awakenings, but actual close encounters with death—produce works of great vision and wisdom and insight and vitality. You become more sensitive to the in-between . . . between life and death, that unhealthy place in the middle, which is neither one nor the other. It is the place I am in right now, and the place I have seen so many times before. Patients who are sick sometimes hover between the two realities. I recall actual events, of real physical sickness, where patients are neither dead nor alive. But since Diagnosis Day I have seen the same in-between state in people who are not sick but who hover in this middle place because they cannot seem to grasp the great gift of life around them. It is that scale I have spoken about before. If white is alive and black is dead, then the grey area in the middle is what I am describing. And that is where I am right now. It is not a pleasant place to be, particularly if you are tending towards the darker shades of grey.

It is getting darker for me now. As I move inexorably towards my own mortality, the scale turns slowly but determinedly towards those darker shades. I will have ups and downs yet, moments where the dial hovers and maybe even shifts a little back in the other direction. But there will come a time when the dial does not spin back at all.

I have spent a decade following a dream, and that dream was to help people move out of this in-between place, to encourage them to grasp hold of life. Half of that decade has been spent trying to give myself the same opportunity, but the dial is about to drop. No more in-between for me.

What comes next is the end.

CHAPTER 12
A much brighter world

We need ugliness in the world in order to appreciate the beauty, and vice versa. It's through my ugliness, my brokenness, that I now appreciate the world in a whole new light. It's my suffering that makes the world that much brighter, that much more colourful, and that much more worth living. It is cancer that has brought a whole new meaning to life, even if that life is much shorter than anticipated.

Conversely, it's the beauty of life that allows me to recognise the ugly: the injustice, the oppression, the suffering, the poverty, the needless loss of life, the insatiable greed for material goods. Recognising this does not empower me to better avoid it, but to better be a part of the solution. I think we instinctively use this recognising ability to avoid the ugly, instead of perhaps being the solution to it. Being the solution to the ugly and the brokenness . . . that's powerful. Or, even better . . . it's beautiful.

'Beautiful and ugly', The Boredom Blog, November 27, 2009

When the iPhone 6 comes out I am going to buy it regardless of whether I am a day out from dying or five, if only because it marks the milestone that I survived long enough to get it. And because Hannah will get a good upgrade when I die. I would also love to get the Apple Watch, but there is not much chance of that.

Early on in my illness, I worried about whether or not I would make it to the New Zealand Rugby World Cup. But I did, and I even attended games. We lived right next to Eden Park at the time, which was great. That was a goal for me, something to survive long enough to see. Another one has been the *Game of Thrones* series on television, but the books have not even been finished yet. I will never find out what happens at the end of that.

I will not be alive for the Cricket World Cup, I know that, but I did see the third in the Batman series, *The Dark Knight Rises*. I was desperate to stay alive long enough for that. I will not be alive long enough to see the new *Star Wars* movie, though. I am not sure if that is a tragedy or not.

———

I travel.

In my imagination, when I can. To places I have been, and to places I have not yet been. I am exhausted now, so there is not much more I can do except think about the places we have explored together, Hannah and I. And then I imagine the places we would have gone. Our hearts were set on adventures that would have taken a lifetime to fulfil. I could not imagine when I saw her there by the fire that she would have the same passion burning in her heart. How wonderful it would have been. What challenges we would have faced. What amazing things we would have achieved together.

———

She is on the bed beside me as I remember our trips together, prodding my memory as it fails.

Elise is here too, playing quietly.

We talk about Italy, Peru, Cambodia, Laos, Vietnam. The food. The people. The things we saw. Stories of ancient civilisations. Incredible meals cooked on the street. The most laid-back people you could ever hope to meet. I can see a track on the hill along which we walked for hours and hours. And we taste the food. I mean, really taste the food.

I am back in Rome with Hannah. It is the month we buy our house. I am still recovering from my second relapse and the hope that was stolen from us. We have talked about children and decided . . . not yet. But very soon.

So here we are in Rome. The Coliseum. The Vatican. All the landmarks. Then down to Pompeii and the Amalfi coast. The train up to Cinque Terre where we meet friends. Then to Milan. From Milan to Venice, Venice to Bologna. We absorb a country when we travel, Hannah and I. We take it all in. A sensory overload so that we never have to go back. 'But Italy was such a cool place,' I say to Hannah. She agrees. 'We would have gone back to Tuscany, for sure,' she says, 'hired a villa and stayed for three weeks . . .'

I wish.

We are in Peru. Tramping in the Andes. And this is something else. We trek for four days and see no one other than the indigenous inhabitants. It is so barren. So amazing. I am on chemo. I have cancer, but we are trekking 4000 metres above the sea. We trek 20 kilometres in a day. Hannah says, 'It felt like you didn't have cancer that whole month.' And I remember. I remember the rage, too. A history of a people destroyed, utterly pillaged. The sort of fight I would have taken on, had I lived. In different parts of the world. Vietnam perhaps. Or parts of Africa.

Now we are in Laos. So laid-back. So relaxed. Before the first relapse, back in the days of 40 per cent. Staying on the Mekong Delta. The most relaxed little town on the banks of the most relaxed river, in the most relaxed country in the world. French all over the place, traces of past colonial days. Laotian cuisine for breakfast, with a baguette.

Now Thailand and Vietnam and Cambodia. We do these with Singapore and the Philippines in the one trip. Vietnam? People who love Vietnam have never been to Cambodia or Laos. It is too easy to get scammed in Vietnam, Hannah reminds me. Cambodia less so. And even less in Laos.

Now I am in India, my least favourite of all. Too pushy, too rude, too much corruption. And I never liked the food. But that is their culture.

But yum, now we are remembering food. Lechón manok in the Philippines—barbecued chicken better than anywhere else in the world. A whole leg on a skewer. And absolutely delicious.

Potatoes and grains in Peru. Nothing to write home about there.

Back in Asia, and pad thai cooked on the street. Delicious.

But Italy. Oh my goodness. The best, I mean the very best, spaghetti carbonara in Rome—by far the best meal of my life. I can taste it even now. So, so delicious. And to eat it where it originated. Just perfect. Follow that up with a degustation menu in a small suburban restaurant on the outskirts of Florence, the most expensive meal we had in Italy. To eat like a local—there is nothing better.

No wonder I put on 3 kilograms in Italy. Every other place we visited, the weight came off. But that carbonara. If anybody serves carbonara with cream in it, tell them they don't know what they are doing. It is just an egg when it is done properly. Crispy pancetta as well. The egg cooks when you put it on the pasta as you serve. The timing has to be perfect. That is where the skill lies. Done right, the egg alone becomes the sauce. Some salt and pepper. The pasta cooked just right.

The best meal ever.

———————

When I am alone, in my thoughts I travel to places I have not yet been. I go to the countries of the world I have not yet seen. I have adventures in my own way, because I will always be a traveller at heart. I have wanted to see most of the world. And most of the world I have not yet visited. In the few glimpses I have had, in the places we have been, I have wanted to see more and more.

I travel to places that are in the news and current affairs. I am not sure why. For example, I travel to the Middle East. That would have been a place we would have seen together, had the trip not been cancelled. I really, really want . . . wanted . . . to get to the Himalayas. Do some tramping and trekking, get to Everest base camp, perhaps—although it has become the tourist thing to do, so maybe not.

I would like to have travelled to Africa. I never got there, despite it being my goal for so long. In some ways our trip to Africa was where this all began—the destination we never reached, a metaphor for my life.

No matter. My imagination takes me there instead.

In my best dreams I travel to the future. It is where I have always spent most of my time, the future—setting goals, shaping dreams, driving towards new possibilities. In my imagination, I can travel through time.

I look up at the stars sometimes and I imagine how, in the future, we will not be limited to travelling on this globe alone. We will travel the stars. We will see other planets. And we will see just how huge the universe is.

We are so small, and so fleeting, despite the drama we attach to our lives. We appear at moments in history then disappear again without so much as recording a blip. The story just rolls along, into a future we cannot possibly imagine. And all around us, space expands beyond measure, to galaxy clusters and super-clusters, in a universe that dwarfs our feeble existence.

We think our lives are so significant, our lives that end in a bed, in a warm room on the upstairs floor of a suburban New Zealand home, about 50 years too soon.

But ours is just a medium-sized sun, after all.

In a solar system on the tip of a spiral galaxy.

Dr Jared Noel
September 24, 2014

EPILOGUE
We are not alone

Jared's heart-on-sleeve-style willingness to speak and blog and share his story with whoever will listen has allowed us an amazing insight into the lives of countless people who have fought cancer, some of whom have lived to tell the tale, others of whom have not. Our lives are richer for meeting these people, for connecting with their families. Though you would never wish the experience on anyone, the knowledge that we are not alone in this is strangely comforting.

This blog began as a distraction, a very real way to pass the time as chemotherapy threatened to drive Jared 'up the wall'. Over time I have observed its function change; it has become a dynamic, relational tool, where Jared interacts with his online community (with you!), family, friends, colleagues, a global village of people who encourage, challenge, reflect and pray. It is a very tangible reminder to us that though we walk a rugged path we did not choose, we are not alone. And for this we are thankful.

Thank you for listening to Jared. Thank you for being there for us.

Hannah.

'Not alone', The Boredom Blog, March 8, 2010

Jared passed away on the morning of Wednesday, October 8, 2014, a full two weeks after working on his story for the final time.

The night before he died, Jared was lying in his hospital bed in our room, peacefully, unconscious. The family had gathered, believing that his time was near. Elise's evening routine was to have her last feed then say goodnight to everyone, including Jared. And it was time for her to say goodbye. I asked the family to leave the three of us for a few minutes and closed the door. And we prayed together as a family, as I have prayed with Elise every night since she was very small.

There, just the three of us in the room where we had spent so much family time in recent weeks, and where Jared had worked so hard to complete the telling of his story for Elise, we asked Jesus to take Daddy to heaven. Because this was what Jared wanted so desperately. Anyone who saw him in those final few days was praying that same prayer—for the ultimate release from his suffering, which was so painfully evident.

It is hard to know whether Jared was ever aware that the three of us were alone in that space at that time, praying that prayer together. Who knows whether he heard us, or perhaps even sensed that, at least from the perspective of the two people who were most dear to him, he was being given permission to go.

He died at 25 minutes past eleven the following morning, surrounded by his family, enveloped in love.

We miss him every day.

———————

Jared loved extravagantly, had an infectious sense of humour, and a profound vision of the greatness he would achieve through following his passion to serve in the undeveloped world.

His tendency to extravagance was nowhere more profoundly expressed than on the day of his marriage proposal to me. His long years of study meant his student loan was excessive, yet Jared's money or lack of it never stopped him doing anything, especially when it came to love.

The engagement story was very important to Jared. I loved the story, and he certainly did it for me, but the amount of joy he got explaining it to people or hearing me recount it was huge. And of course, all his friends were annoyed with him because he set the bar so high for all these younger guys at med school who were not yet married or engaged. And he loved that.

Jared was the flowers-for-no-reason guy. Never on Valentine's Day, though—he would not be dictated to by a foreign culture. When it came to birthdays and Christmases, we would agree how much we would spend and he could never stick to it. He was a top-shelf guy . . . gifts, flowers, Apple products. He loved extravagantly and gave extravagantly, and he got just as much pleasure from that as others did.

One of the things I missed the most in those final few months was Jared's sense of humour. I remember, in his final few weeks, making a joke I fully expected him to laugh at—but his response was, 'That's not funny.' It caused me to stop: I was losing parts of Jared before he was even gone, and his humour, that lightness about him that I knew and loved, was an early casualty.

And yet, I don't need to think too far back to recall moments of real laughter. We have a beautiful video of Elise. It was around late May, during our trip around the North Island visiting family and friends. Elise is about four months old and she is sitting on Jared's knee. One of her cousins, who was about eighteen months at the time, was looking at Elise and laughing. So then she would laugh. Spontaneous laughter was quite new for her at the time. So then the cousin would laugh, then she would laugh. And Jared was just giggling the whole way through it. Elise will enjoy that video one day.

Jared's sense of humour was quite black at times. His colleagues liked to recount moments in the hospital when Jared would make a joke or one-liner relating to his own situation that would be primarily intended to shock people, or at least make them feel incredibly awkward. Colleagues, nurses, bosses, no one was spared. He was really fun. We shared lots of laughter together. But there were fewer moments like that towards the end.

Jared had a vulnerable side, too, for all his confidence and intelligence and conviction, and he uncovered a new level of vulnerability in his last days. When he fell out of bed on his second night home, there was an acute sense of vulnerability that he had not felt in his own home until that point. To need me and my mum to help him back into bed was a blow, a level of embarrassment he had not anticipated. I think he endured a lot of grief associated with that moment.

Some goodbyes were harder than others, too, and Jared made quite a few in our home. How do you say goodbye to your closest friend, knowing full well you will never see him again? The finality of that goodbye rattled Jared—and every day after that was harder. In his 'chemo phase', Jared would always bounce back—the feeling of illness was always temporary—but one of the things he found really hard in those final weeks was accepting that he was not going to get better. The next day was not going to be any better than today, and things were probably going to get worse. He talked about rehab in those last few weeks but also knew there was probably no coming back from how he was feeling.

There were some triumphs, though. When Jared first came home he had no mobility whatsoever. He was stuck in bed.

When they decreased the local anaesthetic on his intrathecal pump, he could get up and bear weight and move around with his walker. He could get downstairs and use his wheelchair—all those things that had actually seemed quite impossible when he first got home. They added significantly to his quality of life in those final weeks. His dream of moving around the house was a small one compared to the dreams he had fought so hard to achieve over the years. But in the context of his final few weeks at home, it was an important contributor to his quality of life.

———————

Jared and I met beside a fire in the Blue Mountains near Sydney one morning before breakfast. He remembers that correctly. Other aspects of the story I know he has interpreted slightly differently to me. And some things he has chosen not to admit.

There was a reasonable Kiwi contingent at the conference, about ten from Auckland, if I recall correctly, with many of whom we remain in touch, as Jared knew them well. Kiwis rose early due to the time difference, and on the third morning of the conference, while I was sitting by the fire, Jared showed up and said, 'Hi, I'm Jared, from Auckland.'

We proceeded to spend the whole of that day together. Jared said later that he would ask me what workshop I was going to, and even if he had not planned to attend that one he would go just to continue this conversation throughout the day. We really covered a lot of stuff pretty quickly. I had been on my medical elective to Nepal and was probably still riding the wave of potential in the career I had chosen. I came to the conference with recent experience and a passion for medical mission in the developing world. Jared clearly had that as well. That was the substance of that first conversation—how he'd had these experiences in the Philippines and had wanted to do medicine to further that. We had a lot in common. And that is what that first conversation was, connecting with each other in that area of calling and vision.

It was during this first conversation, too, that Jared talked about feeling called to greatness of some kind. It sounds a bit arrogant to say that now, but it did not come across that way at the time. He just clearly knew he was destined to have an impact on the world. By the end of the day, the two of us realised, independently, that something significant had happened. We were walking back to where we were staying that night. And this sounds so cheesy now, but a shooting star went across the sky. And I remember Jared saying to me much later that he felt, in that moment, that it would be the most natural thing in the world to just grab my hand.

But he didn't do it, he said, because that would have been weird.

There is a part of me that thinks that if cancer had never entered the picture, Jared and I together could have done so much more. I know he has done enormous things in the time he has battled cancer. He really has lived an extraordinary life in the context of his illness. And so if there is any part of me that wishes it never happened, there is so much more of me that sees the extraordinary man Jared was in the way he chose to live with his illness, and in the way he chose to communicate that to the world. That really quietens the part of me that grieves at that sense of lost opportunity.

I have been a supporting actress in Jared's remarkable story. A lot of people say to me, 'Behind every great man . . .' But I do not think I have been a huge influence on the way Jared has chosen to navigate his illness. I think I have supported him in that and given him some strength to be able to keep going and do the things he has done. Fighting cancer has been something we have done together, but he is the one who chose to be so honest and out-there with his story. It was a decision he took alone. He wanted to let the world in on his experiences in order to let his story help others in their own struggles. That took enormous courage and trust.

I know that Jared accepted the mantle of antihero as an appropriate way to describe the unique role he played, but in many eyes, not least mine, he was a true hero. And he did achieve greatness. Maybe not in the way we envisaged we would together, but in a way that influenced and encouraged many people.

By the time of his funeral, the views of Jared's blog were almost three-quarters of a million. On the day of his death, it was viewed more than 45,000 times by 18,000 different people. A year before, in the same month the Givealittle campaign was running, his blog was viewed almost 90,000 times by more than 31,000 visitors. In the 30 days surrounding Jared's death and funeral, there were almost 95,000 views from New Zealand alone, more than 13,000 from Australia, 4000 from the United States, 400 from the United Kingdom, and 1200 from Canada. This was as well as speaking to thousands of people at events over the period of his sickness.

I think it is fair to say that Jared achieved a measure of the greatness to which he always believed he had been called.

None of this stopped him feeling guilty about what cancer had taken from us and from our future together. When he said this to me, I would tell him that it was not his fault and he would say how unhelpful that was, because he still felt that way. But I think what he felt was sorry, not in an apologetic way, but in a regretful way. I think it comes down to lost opportunities rather than regret. We both felt that way.

It was eighteen months from meeting Jared to getting married, then eleven months from getting married to when he was diagnosed with cancer, so far more of our time together was with cancer than without. We lived with this for a long time, relative to that short period when we were young and dreaming and had all these plans to do great things together. And then the game changed the night Jared had surgery. I have long reconciled to myself that our life from that moment was never going to be the one we had planned.

So many things contributed to changing the vision we had when we first set out on this journey together. Every time the game changed, from diagnosis to first relapse then surgery then second relapse—each moment remains vivid in my memory. I find myself going back there, remembering how I felt and how Jared responded and what we did. They are moments in time that are frozen and help me recall key parts of the story.

Elise was also a game changer—I think the arrival of children results in a shift in priorities for most people. In many ways she made dying so much harder for Jared—but in the best possible way. Suddenly he had so much to live for . . . and so much more to miss out on. As for the future, we have lived for the past six years in a constant state of uncertainty, unable to plan our lives more than three to six months in advance. That is highly challenging for a type A person like me, who likes to have a five-year plan!

Jared has said to me to go wherever, to do whatever. I think he ultimately trusted me to make those decisions and was very careful not to constrain me in any way. You can carry a great burden of expectation—even from someone you have loved and journeyed with—if they set any limits on what you do after they have gone. Jared has been very gracious in that way. I think he would like to know that at some point I would take Elise to the developing world and travel reasonably widely with her. That was something that was important to us both.

Do I see myself in five or ten years doing the thing Jared and I set out to do when we got married? It is complicated. I find myself looking at a future without Jared, who was so bound up in that initial vision and dream that it is hard for me to imagine how it would be without him. And having a child wholly dependent on me does not make it easy to go off to Sierra Leone on a whim. Elise will, from now on, always frame how I weigh up risk. It is not that I cannot do any of the things Jared and I talked about, but the future without him looks very different.

This is a new beginning, but one that is very rich with history, legacy and purpose.

———————

A week after the final session of working on his story, Jared was downstairs in a wheelchair. This was the Wednesday, a full week before he died. Even so close to the end he was still coming down, going out into the garden and looking around—noting the ever-increasing height of his beloved pittosporums and bemoaning the way neighbourhood cats and birds would scatter woodchips into the grass. In the evenings we were still watching *My Kitchen Rules*, but Jared was finding it increasingly difficult to follow what was happening even in a simple television program. It seemed that this confused state heralded the beginning of the end.

The marked deterioration was over the period of a week, and at the end, Jared was unconscious for a day and a half. For a man of so many words, communication was sporadic in those final days. There were no final words, no last-minute deathbed proclamations. I think the last thing Jared actually said to me was, 'Can you put the bed up?' In the days leading up to his death, there was a lot of sleeping and he became increasingly confused, finding it more and more difficult to follow a conversation; even getting an answer from him to a direct question was quite hard. There were times when he was clearly uncomfortable but it was hard to know whether it was terminal agitation or whether he was in pain. I would ask him at those times whether he wanted pain relief, and he really struggled to say either yes or no.

There are certain signs that accompany terminal illness in the final stages. What Jared was going through before the end was not surprising to the hospice people. He would get anxious for no apparent reason. He would pluck at the air and adopt strange postures that were not obviously pain but were clearly discomfort. He required a lot of pain relief and anti-anxiety medication over those last few days. I did not want him lying there in a state of either pain or agitation and not being able to communicate that or get relief from it. It is like having a small baby—reading the signs as best you can, trying to anticipate discomfort when communication is limited and do your best to alleviate it.

It was clear over that final week that Jared's death was imminent. His parents stayed with us for the last few nights, bunking down in the study. The night before he died Jared's mum gathered the immediate family around, his brother and sister and their partners. My mum had been there for months, her role primarily to help me care for Elise—I could not have coped without her.

So the family gathered, ate dinner, talked in hushed tones, cried and prayed. Jared was unable to engage in it at all but he was probably aware of being surrounded. The following morning, nothing had changed greatly. He was clearly in renal (kidney) failure. There did not seem to be much of a deterioration overnight, but as I looked more closely at him I mentally cancelled my plan to pop out to the supermarket—it did not seem like the right thing to leave the house that morning.

His mum, Ruth, and I were sitting with Jared. She left the room to make a phone call and all of a sudden his breathing changed, quite significantly. I took his pulse and it was 30 or 40 beats a minute. It was clear to both Ruth and me that he had minutes left. He was gasping but not distressed. I sat weeping at his bedside. His sister arrived in time to see Jared take his last breath.

From the moment Jared's breathing changed to witnessing his last breath took about ten minutes. It was fast, and I think that was good. Had it happened in the middle of the night I am not sure that I would have woken up.

So, with little fight, and with little noise, Jared was gone.

I am so relieved that Jared has been released from his suffering. And so incredibly proud of the life he lived, which has spoken such volumes to so many people in the way he navigated his course and shared his suffering and his hope with the world. I think what will come later is the inevitable loneliness and missing everything he was in my life, but I am just so relieved for him that those dark and difficult days of waiting for the end have passed. It was very clear to me, as soon as he died, that his spirit was gone. I looked at his face and he was just different. We had said our goodbyes.

There is a photo taken of Jared, Elise and me on the day he stopped working on his story. It was the last photo taken of us as a family, and is the last image taken of Jared. For many of the people who knew Jared, it will remain the last image they have of him. He had withdrawn from his wider friends and acquaintances right down to family in the end, and was not updating his blog, but on the day before he died, several friends posted on his Facebook wall to ask how he was going. It was strange that so many seemed to be thinking of him on that particular day. Perhaps they realised without even being told that he was at death's door.

Jared was ready to go weeks before he died, but why his body held on for far longer than his mind or his spirit wanted to was a mystery to him. He woke up the Sunday before the Wednesday he died and said to me, 'Why am I still alive?' I did not have an answer for him. There was very little quality to his life by that stage, and I know that was where the question came from. It seemed so pointless that he should have to get through the days. Mercifully, within 48 hours of saying that, he lapsed into unconsciousness.

It broke my heart, watching Jared over those final days and weeks, facing that very imminent mortality while being at a loss to do anything about it. While the inevitability of death is true for all of us, not all experience the pain of the body holding on, long after the mind and spirit are ready to leave this world.

This was a guy who had stood in front of thousands of people and said, 'I'm okay with dying.' What about when you are not okay with dying? What do we make of that? Were you lying when you said that to all those people? Or is death harder than any of us can ever conceive of when we are well? Jared had great sadness in his final days, something I had never seen in him, not to that extent. And why would he not? He was losing everything—the ability to engage, to enjoy, to contribute. One by one, he lost all of those things. All of the quality of life he had fought to maintain, even the simple pleasures of home, all of these things were taken away from him. This is the heart-breaking reality of dying, something even the best palliative care falls short of fixing.

I have peace about Jared dying. I have no regrets, any more than Jared did. Between the two of us there was nothing left unsaid. We worked really hard at keeping short accounts in those final months—of being so open and honest with each other that Jared would feel free to go when it was his time, and I would not have to live long term with unnecessary guilt or pain.

There was no notable final conversation, but Jared told me a great many times in those days, even when he was confused, that he loved me. He was very un-confused about that point. Within that final week, in a moment when he was slightly agitated, he said, 'I love you, Hannah Noel. I love you, Hannah Noel.' It seemed strange that Jared would use my first name and surname in the same sentence, but he was saying it purpose-fully, urgently, as if he knew that his last battle would be against incoherence. Like anything Jared ever communicated, to me or to the thousands of people who followed his writing or heard him speak in front of massive crowds, he wanted to be very clear. I think he knew that it would not be long before he was unable to say those words to me again.

Before Jared died, he did manage to achieve one final mile-stone. He held on long enough to hold the iPhone 6.

And he very much approved.

Dr Hannah Noel
October 2014

Acknowledgements

It's 28 August 2014, and I enter the Noel home for the first time.

It is clean and bright, the breeze is allowed to blow through, and the bright walls and open plan living areas create a generous sense of space, air and life. It is very much the type of home I would expect two young doctors to make.

There is a baby in the house too—Elise. On this first day she is sitting upright in her chair beside the dining table, with chubby, flushed cheeks and sparkling, intelligent eyes. Present, animated and expectant. And quite ignorant of the reason behind all the activity going on around her.

This does not feel like a young man's final resting place. There are no hospital odours, no tears, no gloomy shadows caused by drawn curtains. There are plenty of medicines on top of the dresser, and there's a drip bag hanging from a stand beside Jared's bed which feeds into his side—but the light airiness of the room seems to burn these elements from the scene. This feels like a young couple's marital home. It's a home that anticipates a future. There are rooms for more kids, space for more activity, places for more books on the shelves. There are framed family portraits on the walls. Items of wedding memorabilia placed carefully in the bedroom, the family room, the upstairs lounge. And there are several pairs of shoes in the hallway behind the front door.

I stand undone at these shoes the very first time I see them, unsure whether I'm meant to take mine off as well. Mostly though I am undone by the fact Jared is not there at the front door to greet me. It's been two days since I saw him in the hospice, but I have forgotten already that he is bedridden, that the muscles in his legs have become pretty much ineffective. I notice that none of these shoes are his—that they belong, most likely, to Hannah, or her mother, or Jared's parents—all of whom are there, on this first occasion, to greet me in the doorway with bare or stockinged feet.

I recall this scene because without this group of people this book would not have been possible. And to meet them all in one go like this was like being introduced to the principle characters of Jared's life story right before his narration began. Over the ensuing weeks I observed as they all cared for and upheld one another, and made it possible for Jared to battle his mounting fatigue and sickness in order to complete our interviews. And then when the manuscript was finished they each faced the emotionally arduous task of reliving the story in order to proof the text, without complaint. So, to Hannah's parents, Frances and Sandy, and to Jared's parents, Royston and Ruth, a great deal of thanks is owed for their patience and grace, for creating the space for Jared and I to talk, and for their ongoing support of the project. And to Hannah . . . there aren't words to describe my appreciation of the work she has contributed to this book. In the weeks leading up to Jared's final days, and then afterwards, during many more interviews, and more rounds of proofing and editing, Hannah showed absolute commitment to Jared's story being told authentically and accurately, despite the personal challenges the process created for her. She is a person of immense strength and humility whose heart is all over this book.

Another visitor to the house in those weeks was Nigel Cottle, the 'closest friend' that Jared refers to in the chapter,

'Every Moment Counts'. It was Nigel who brought Jared and me together, just three days before our first conversation on 28 August. Nigel was as passionate as Jared for his story to be told, and was aware that I was looking for a project. How much faith he had that Jared and I could pull it off, I'm not sure. But I am very grateful for his foresight, and for his ongoing friendship.

This project has been bittersweet from the beginning, and one of the biggest regrets I have is that Jared was not able to experience the support, care and professionalism of the team at Allen & Unwin, particularly that of Publisher Jenny Helen, in Auckland, and Senior Editor Sarah Baker, in Sydney. In my final conversation with Jared he told me that he would have loved to have seen the book through to publication, and I know that he would have enjoyed and appreciated A&U's attention to every word, every piece of design and every aspect of publishing strategy around the release of the book. A&U's belief in the story and their passion and thoroughness during the whole process have honoured Jared's memory in the best possible way.

Finally, to Jared himself. What can you say about a guy who, in the final weeks of his life, entrusts his story to a stranger and spends precious, fleeting hours making sure that story will be rich and inspiring. Jared was an extraordinary man, and I was privileged and honoured to be with him at some very precious moments. I felt like a trespasser for most of them, not because of anything Jared said or did but because the final resting place of anyone is sacred ground, and there are countless others who would have been far more deserving of being there with him at those times. Even so, that he invited me into that place in his final days left me feeling profoundly blessed—something I know others have experienced in response to Jared. More than anything, I hope this comes through in the final text.

Writers often have an assumed reader, someone they imagine reading their words and authenticating their writing process. I realised my assumed reader was Jared all along when it hit me that he would never read the book we had worked on together. So, the project has ended but it feels unfulfilled—and always will. But that's the reality of death, and I am deeply, deeply indebted to Jared for letting me experience it the way that I have. As Jared says in the book, there is nothing like confronting mortality—or what it takes from us—to make you appreciate the life you have and the people you have been given to share it with.

If readers experience something of this because of Jared's story, then his hope for this book will have been realised.

David W. Williams

About the author

David Wyn Williams, PhD, is a writer and academic who is published as a journalist and as a theologian. His first book, *This Little Piggy Stayed Home: Barlow, Chambers and the Mafia*, was published in Australia in 1989. He lives and works in Auckland, New Zealand.

Twitter: @davidwilliamsnz
Web: www.davidwwilliams.nz